Health is Wealth

MAKE A DELICIOUS INVESTMENT IN YOU!

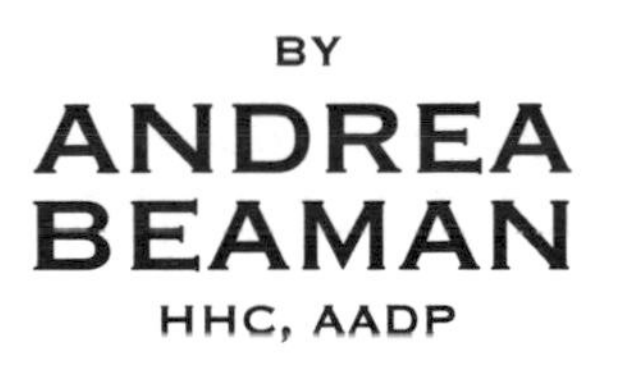

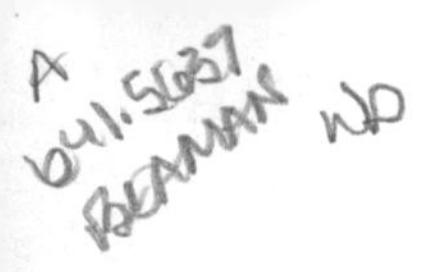

www.AndreaBeaman.com
email: AndreaBeaman@aol.com

Published by Andrea Beaman, New York City

The material contained in Health is Wealth is for general information and the purpose of educating individuals on nutrition, lifestyle, health & fitness and related topics. Should you have any health care related questions, please consult with your physician or other health care provider before embarking on a new treatment, diet, fitness or exercise program.

Cover design Julie Mueller
jam graphics & design, llc

ACKNOWLEGEMENTS 1
INTRODUCTION 3

Chapter 1
MAKING A WISE INVESTMENT 5

Chapter 2
BACK TO THE BASICS 11

Chapter 3
PUT YOUR MONEY WHERE YOUR MOUTH IS! 27

Chapter 4
THIS LITTLE PIGGY WENT TO THE MARKET 34

Chapter 5
PURCHASING THE ESSENTIALS 54

Chapter 6
SAVE BIG BUCKS! 65

Chapter 7
FROM PORRIDGE TO PROSPERITY 74

RECIPES
BREAKFAST PORRIDGE 80
CONGEE 82
MISO SALMON SOUP 83
OATS & ALMONDS 84
SAVORY OATS & SAUSAGE 85
RAVISHING ROLLED OATS 86
POACHED EGGS 88
SCRAMBLED EGGS CON VEGGIES 90
CREAMY POLENTA AND FRIED EGGS 92

Chapter 8

INVESTING IN GOOD STOCK 93

RECIPES

BASIC CHICKEN STOCK 98
DUCK STOCK 99
TURKEY STOCK 100
BEEF STOCK 101
BASIC VEGETABLE STOCK 102
SLOW COOKER STOCK 103

Chapter 9

MEALS THAT WORK! 104

MENU PLAN #1

BLACK-EYED PEAS WITH CHORIZO 112
BASIC BROWN RICE 114
SAVORY RICE & OATS PORRIDGE 114
BRAISED RED CABBAGE AND KALE 115
WINTER COBBLER 116
BLACK-EYED PEA SOUP 118
SAUTÉED BLACK-EYED PEAS AND VEGETABLE WRAP 119
QUICK-COOKING FRIED RICE 120

MENU PLAN #2

SESAME-CRUSTED SOLE 124
SIMPLE SOBA NOODLES 126
SAUTÉED BOK CHOY & CARROTS 127
SOBA NOODLE STIR-FRY 128
FIVE-MINUTE MISO SOUP 129

MENU PLAN #3

BAKED CHICKEN & ROSEMARY-ROASTED POTATOES 133
SIMPLE SAUTÉED CARROTS AND BROCCOLI 134
CHICKEN LIVER PÂTÉ 135
CHEESE AND VEGGIE OMELET 136
HOMEY HOME FRIES 137
QUICK-COOKING CHICKEN CACCIATORE 138
WHOLE GRAIN HERBED GARLIC BREAD 139
CURRIED CHICKEN SALAD 140

WHITE BEAN AND KALE SOUP 141
CRISPY GARLIC CROUTONS 142

MENU PLAN #4
LENTILS WITH SAUTÉED LEEKS, SPINACH, AND SAUSAGE 145
SIMPLE BROWN BASMATI RICE 146
STEAMED WINTER VEGETABLES 147
CRANBERRY DRESSING 148
ROASTING & TOASTING NUTS 149
LENTIL AND VEGETABLE WRAP 150
STIR-FRIED SHRIMP, RICE, AND VEGETABLES 151
SILKY LENTIL SOUP 152
CREAMY COCONUT RICE PUDDING 153

MENU PLAN #5
BASIC BLACK BEANS 156
POLENTA WITH TURKEY SAUSAGE 157
FRIED POLENTA SQUARES 158
SEASONAL BEAN SALAD IN LETTUCE CUPS 159
SPICY BLACK BEAN SOUP WITH POLENTA CROUTONS 160

MENU PLAN #6
WHOLE GRAIN COUSCOUS WITH DRIED CRANBERRIES 163
ROASTED TURKEY WITH HERBED GRAVY 164
SAVORY COUSCOUS PORRIDGE 166
SAUTÉED COLLARD GREENS WITH GARLIC 167
TURKEY AND PASTA SALAD 168
HOMEMADE MAYO 169
CREAMY TURKEY CHOWDER 170
HOT OPENED TURKEY SANDWICHES WITH HERBED GRAVY 171

MENU PLAN #7
TAHINI NOODLES & BRAISED DUCK 174
RENDERED DUCK FAT 175
DUCK BREAST & CHINESE CABBAGE SALAD WITH CRACKLINS 176
HEARTY ROASTED WINTER ROOTS 178
SAUTÉED BRUSSELS SPROUTS WITH CRANBERRIES 179
SAVORY SHIITAKE MUSHROOM SOUP 180
DUCK LIVER PÂTÉ 181
CARAMELIZED ONION SOUP 182

Chapter 10

THE POT OF GOLD 183

RECIPES

MAGNIFICENT MINESTRONG! 186
HEARTY LENTIL STEW 188
SAVORY TURKEY CHILI 190
ONE-POT WILD SALMON STEW 192
SEA BASS SOUP WITH SOBA NOODLES 194
WINTER WHITE BEAN STEW 195
CHUNKY CHICKEN SOUP 196
SUMMER VEGETABLES AND BEAN STEW 197
TEX-MEX CHILI CON CARNE 198
BUFFALO CHILI 200
HEARTY BEEF STEW 202
STEWED LAMB WITH APRICOTS 204

Chapter 11

FROZEN ASSETS 205

RECIPES

CREAMY ASPARAGUS SOUP 208
SPRING PEA SOUP 209
SILKY CORN CHOWDER 210
MIXED VEGETABLE MEDLEY SOUP 211
LENTILS WITH SPINACH AND SAUSAGE 212
NOT SO CHILLY CHILI 213
DELUXE BURGERS 214
SASSY SHRIMP & VEGETABLE STIR FRY WITH NOODLES 215
SIMPLE BERRY SORBETS 216
PEACHES AND CREAM 217

Chapter 12

LIFESTYLE STRATEGIES OF THE HEALTHY & FABULOUS! 218
FOOD RESOURCES 227
ANDREA BEAMAN BOOKS AND PRODUCTS 229
RECIPE INDEX 231

To my Dad, Richard E. Beaman
my biggest fan

ACKNOWLEDGMENTS

Over the past decade, I have listened to clients, students, and fans to learn where they needed assistance incorporating diet and lifestyle improvements into their everyday lives. My deepest thanks to you all. If you hadn't asked so many important questions, we wouldn't have this book. Also, thanks for letting me test recipes on you in my cooking classes. You were truly a captivated audience. Or is that a "captured audience"? Once you were inside my apartment, I wouldn't let you out!

Thank you, Joshua Rosenthal and the Institute for Integrative Nutrition, for encouraging me to share my voice with the world. I'll keep shouting out a message of health; eventually, it will be heard all around the world.

Big thanks to Paula Jacobson and Sheilah Kaufman for their tireless tag-team editing. You two gals are awesome. Thank you, MacKenzie Carpenter, for finding these two gems! MacKenzie traveled via the web, all the way to Maryland, to locate the best editors for this project.

Thank you, Rena Unger, for being the hardest working sous chef in the business and a fantastic support system. Thanks to Jackie Davidson, the newest member of team-beam! Thank you, Donna Sonkin, for your sage advice on hiring a great photographer for the book cover and for being a loyal and loving friend. Thank you, Valerie Feder, for all of your love and support, and for helping me get out into the world in a newsworthy way. You gals are the best!

Thank you, Jordan Matter, for a pretty darn amazing book cover photo. And thank you, Mira Zaki, for my favorite chef headshot. Julie Mueller at Jam Graphics and Design -- I love all of my book covers and everything you have created for me.

Thanks to my family for their love and their support of my career and life choices. A special thank you to my nephews, who are always willing to experiment in the kitchen with me. I totally love you guys.

To all of the farmers and food suppliers who are growing and producing great quality food – thank you! Where there is food, there is life.

Last, but certainly not least, thank you, Pablo Garcia, for nourishing my heart and soul. And for making the most delicious breakfasts so I could finish writing and editing this book. Gracias, Mielo.

INTRODUCTION

Throughout the years of counseling clients about health and diet, I've heard many excuses repeated over and over again: making, eating, or choosing better food is impossible due to demanding work schedules, traveling, no time to cook, eating fast food on the run, dining out with clients, or family gatherings, and social functions that seem to get in the way of good food choices. These excuses may be legitimate, but there are also many simple ways to ensure better health. And that is what I do best -- make a wholesome and nourishing diet and lifestyle work within the modern-day fast-paced society we live in.

Clients are often amazed when I tell them I regularly eat out in restaurants, have an extensive travel schedule, attend social gatherings, and even savor summer barbecues. Everywhere I go, I simply take my food knowledge with me; and with that knowledge, I can create the most delicious and nutritious meals anywhere and at any time – even if I'm stranded in an airport!

I wrote this book to teach you how to get the best foods into your life in the easiest ways possible. Consistently eating better food ensures you are filling up your vitamin and mineral bank and making solid investments in the health of your body. It's imperative we begin investing in our health at the earliest possible time to help prevent future illness. Prevention is the key to long-lasting health.

As you read through this guide, you will learn where to shop, and how to save money, make the most of your time in the kitchen, cook meals in quantity for future use, and stock up and organize the pantry.

You will also learn how to strategize menus to make the most of meals, how to eat out at social functions, what to do around the holidays, and much more. This book can guide you toward ditching some of those lame excuses about why you can't possibly care for yourself, and help you get down to the real business of creating a healthy body and mind.

For many people, taking on their health and eating better can seem like a daunting, expensive, and time-consuming task, but have no fear… I can teach you how to nourish yourself with the best food money can buy even if you're on a tight budget. Remember -- you are worth every penny you invest in yourself and in your health.

Wishing you vibrant health,
Andrea Beaman, HHC, CHEF, AADP

Chapter 1

MAKING A WISE INVESTMENT

In the modern-day rat race, while striving to achieve financial success, or just plain trying to keep up with the darn Joneses (Who the heck are the Joneses anyway?), we have literally run ourselves ragged. We spend long hours at the office, eat fast food and junk food, or skip meals altogether. We also lack daily physical exercise, sunshine, and adequate sleep. All of these detrimental lifestyle behaviors are negatively affecting our health.

According to government statistics, we spend billions of our hard-earned bucks on diseases *directly caused* by a nutrient-deficient diet and unhealthy lifestyle. Obesity, cancer, diabetes, heart disease, depression, infertility, osteoporosis, and other illnesses are literally eating away the money we've worked so tediously to amass.[1]

Our current lifestyle model doesn't make sense. We are working ourselves into a state of physical and emotional sickness -- for what? So we can have a better life *after* we retire? We cannot enjoy retirement if we can't even get out of bed because our bodies have physically failed us; or, more appropriately, because we have failed our bodies.

Today's skyrocketing rates of disease could possibly have been avoided had we been taught the fundamentals of food at an early age, just as we are taught reading, writing, and arithmetic. Attending school

---

1 http://www.ars.usda.gov/research/programs/programs.htm?docid=400&npnumber=107

trains the mind, preparing us for the workforce. As a child I was taught two plus two equals four over and over again until I *got it*. And, if I didn't *get it,* I couldn't move up to the next grade level. It was that simple. I would have been left behind or forced to attend summer school until those facts and figures were ingrained in my mind, and I could recite them backwards, forwards, and upside down.

I believe, had we been similarly taught about food choices and how they relate to the health and maintenance of the body, preventing or healing illness could be as easy for us as two plus two equals four. But, for some reason food theory and preparation aren't on the agenda at most schools. Actually, that's not entirely true. I remember sitting through mandatory home economics class in high school. It was there I learned how to make a sticky sweet cinnamon roll. The students were given store-bought dough and told to spread it flat on the table until it resembled a square Sicilian pizza crust. We were instructed to coat the raw dough with softened butter, ground cinnamon, and lots of sugar. Lastly, we rolled the dough into a log-shaped object and baked it at 350° F for 20 minutes. Voila...cinnamon roll! That was the extent of my training in food preparation. And, it seems quite possible that everyone in the USA was given that very same home economics class and it could be the reason for our current health crisis! As impressionable youngsters, we were taught two great lessons: two plus two equals four and how to prepare sweet cinnamon rolls.

Wholesome, nutritious food should be at the core of our eating instincts, but it's not. Somehow we've either lost touch with that basic knowledge or were never taught it in the first place. And, in our haste to make top dollars, or keep up with the rising cost of living, we've neglected this most primal instinct for ourselves and for our children.

The theme of this book is clear: choose pure, simple ingredients including whole grains, beans, animal proteins, vegetables, fruits, nuts and seeds, and fats, like those our ancestors ate. You may have heard this a million times, and you'll hear it repeated over and over until it finally hits home and you *get it* -- like a mom asking her child to brush his teeth before bed. The kid usually complains and has to be told every night until he finally gets it, and the simple act of brushing the teeth becomes a habit. That's what I want to instill in you. The more you consistently prepare and eat the best quality foods, the more this action becomes a healthy habit that you eventually won't even think about. It'll just happen automatically.

Throughout the years, I've heard clients fault demanding work schedules for eating on the run, skipping meals entirely, or over-stimulating themselves with coffee, sugar, and those blasted cinnamon rolls! Others dine out on a regular basis and do not *know* how to order healthfully in a restaurant. Some mention family gatherings, social functions, and various other daily activities that get in the way of making wise food and lifestyle choices. These reasons for eating poorly are understandable, especially since we haven't been taught the basics of how to make the most of our time in the kitchen or how to make the best choices when we're out and about taking care of our daily business.

I'm not going to sugarcoat it: wholesome food does take some effort to purchase and prepare, and most people either do not have time to spare or refuse to make it a priority. Many of us are overburdened with responsibilities and work commitments and are too exhausted to invest the time or energy needed to properly nourish ourselves.

What people may not realize is that there are quick and easy ways to get better food into their lives without spending hours slaving over a hot stove. With a little food knowledge and lifestyle savvy, it's possible to make the best food choices while out in the world, too. From practical wisdom and first-hand experience, I have included information in this book that can teach you how to get the best quality foods into your life and into your body as quickly, easily, and painlessly as possible, without disrupting a busy schedule. Thank goodness for that! You can enjoy a nourishing breakfast and still make it to the board meeting on time. Whew!

This book does not reveal any trendy new diet revelation (Do we really need another fad diet?), hold the secret to the fountain of youth, or teach you how to live forever. Our lives are finite. That's a bummer, I know. Death is an inevitable part of this life; but we don't have to get to the end of it crawling, limping, or being wheeled there with one kidney, half a liver, and a monkey's heart because we've neglected to eat well and properly nourish ourselves while trying to make ends meet.

The human body, perfect in its design, can remain intact, strong, and fit until the very last breath *if* we learn how to invest in the best food and lifestyle choices as often as possible.

There is no need to quit your job and run off into the mountains seeking solitude in a cave to improve your health – although it may help, and I would highly recommend this as an option for some folks. Vibrant health begins first and foremost with one of our most basic needs: food. All creatures on this planet need to eat to live. As humans, sitting at the top of the food chain, we have a wide variety of food choices when it comes to finding our next meal. Unfortunately, having so many choices has also become one of our biggest problems. In fact, there is so much unhealthful food on the market disguised as "health food" that we don't know what the heck to eat. Have no fear -- we'll cut through the "organic" baloney and get to the nourishing nuggets of wisdom.

The quality of our food impacts our energy levels, health status, and essentially our overall existence. There is a multitude of scientific information proving the connection between eating better quality food and experiencing better health. Many people already know this, but fall short in incorporating the practical information into their daily lives. Or, all too often, people will wait until their vitamin and mineral reserves are completely depleted and sickness has consumed them before they opt to make improvements.

That's what I did. I waited for the illness to knock me to the floor before I made the necessary changes. I was a stimulant-addicted junk-food-junkie and chronic dieter. My nutritional deficiencies showed up in the form of thyroid disease and poor immunity. For other people it may show up as some form of cancer, heart disease, diabetes, arthritis, infertility, autoimmune disease, or any other ailment. If the body is subsisting on cinnamon rolls and stimulants and isn't getting adequate nutrition to function properly, it won't. Waiting for sickness to come isn't the smartest thing to do because rebounding from illness takes much more time and energy than keeping the body healthy in the first place.

"Health is wealth" literally means it's possible to have a rich life without compromising ourselves in the process. Don't get me wrong --

earning millions of dollars could certainly help make eating well and living healthfully a heck of a lot easier! But in the long run, spending our money trying to *reclaim* health after it's been *ruined* can completely deplete our retirement funds.

We need to learn how to invest in our health on a daily basis. So, it's back to the basics to learn the ABCs and 123s of wholesome and delicious food to improve health on every level. Put on your thinking caps (and your aprons), and let's get started!

Chapter 2

BACK TO THE BASICS

Before you begin shopping, cooking, and investing in health, it's important to have a basic idea of how much food you and your family *could* eat at any given meal. We've all heard the expression, "eat a fully balanced meal," but what exactly does that mean? According to the United States Department of Agriculture's (USDA) *MyPyramid.gov,* a balanced meal consists of grains, vegetables, fruits, milk, meat, beans, and fats. That is a wide variety of food that supports many facets of the food industry, but how much are we supposed to eat? Following directions on the government's website, I entered my stats: height (5'4" on a tall day), weight (128 pounds, usually) and daily exercise activity level (30 to 60 minutes). I was redirected to my own personal pyramid recommending 2,000 calories per day. I haven't counted calories since I stopped "dieting" over a decade ago, so I had no idea what 2,000 calories a day might look like or taste like.

Curious to discover how many calories it is that I *do* consume on a daily basis, I entered the food eaten on that particular day: a slice of multi-grain bread smeared with grass-fed butter topped with one poached egg for breakfast; a handful of trail mix consisting of roasted nuts and dried fruit as a midmorning snack; brown rice pilaf with a small thigh of stewed chicken (about 3 to 4 ounces) and tomatoes, baby mesclun greens topped with a few tablespoonfuls of black beans and corn salad for lunch; a ripe juicy peach in the late afternoon for a snack; and pan-seared salmon (about 4 to 5 ounces) with sautéed summer vegetables for dinner.

Oh… and I almost forgot. I also indulged in a sinful oatmeal walnut raisin cookie that was the size of my head! Just joshin' ya. The cookie was about the size of my palm. My day was delicious and fully satisfying but, according to the *MyPyramid.gov* calorie counter, my intake for the day was a mere 1561 calories. That was 439 calories *fewer* than what I should have been eating.

The *MyPyramid.gov* menu planner suggested I wasn't eating enough calories and needed to increase dairy, fruit, and good fats to help reach my 2,000-calorie-per-day goal. According to their recommendation, I was to:

- Choose a **fat-free** or **low-fat** yogurt for a snack
- Have a cappuccino or latte with **fat-free** milk
- Use **fat-free** or **low-fat** milk instead of water in oatmeal and hot cereal
- Make a smoothie in the blender from fruit and **low-fat** or **fat-free** yogurt
- For dessert, make pudding with **fat-free** or **low-fat** milk
- Top casseroles with **low-fat** or **fat-free** cheese
- Use **fat-free** or **low-fat** milk when making cream of tomato or mushroom soup

Do you see a trend here? *MyPyramid.gov* planner suggested all low-fat and fat-free dairy options. I do *not* eat fat-free or low-fat anything! As a former dieter, I know neglecting fat can trigger cravings for excess carbohydrates and sweet sugary snacks. And all that sugar inevitably turns into fat and gets stored in my body. I also know my body needs all of the fat in those dairy products to absorb the beneficial nutrients such as the fat-soluble vitamins and minerals that lie within. Besides, I think dairy food without the fatty luscious creamy texture tastes pretty darn horrible. Spit, spit, pattooey! One important thing to remember as you begin getting to know food is... fat equals flavor. Eating full-fat products supports and satisfies the body (and the taste-buds, too); just eat a smaller quantity.

However, let's get back to the infamous food pyramid. The daily three cups of dairy recommended by the government would certainly increase my caloric intake and my body weight at the same time. I don't believe that amount of milk and milk products are beneficial to my adult health. Babies drink milk, and I am not a baby (wahhhhhhhh!). I do eat small quantities of butter, yogurt, and cheese, but certainly *not* three cups daily.

According to Walter Willett, Professor of Nutrition at Harvard University School of Public Health, the USDA food pyramid is biased by the interests of big agribusiness industries. "There's an inherent problem with the USDA creating the pyramid. The economic interests are so strong — and beef and dairy are the most powerful — that I think it's impossible for the USDA to say that people should limit red meat consumption or limit dairy products to one or two servings a day. It's very difficult for them to be objective, so it's probably the worst possible agency to do the pyramid."[2]

Without adding what we can assume is the *biased* amount of recommended dairy products into my diet, I returned to the menu planner and entered a few more days of my usual *summer* eating habits. The

---

2 http://www.intelihealth.com/IH/ihtIH/WSANP000/325/28910/328885.html?d=dmtContent

results all came back around 1,600 calories. I figured this was the correct amount of calories to be eating at that time of year because both my health and weight are excellent. My weight is ideal for my height; I am not undernourished (skinny) or "overnourished" (overweight). Furthermore, my bones are strong, all internal systems are functioning normally, and my energy levels are good.

Changing gears, I entered the food I would normally consume on a cold, snowy, wintry day in New York City. I increased food intake in all categories, plus added some hearty stews and more fat into my meal plan. I'm generally hungrier in the winter (craving more meat and fat) as my body literally requires additional fuel to keep me warm and insulated. Calories generate heat. I usually gain 5 to 7 pounds during the cold winter months, but it's *not* an unhealthy weight. It's my body's way of protecting me from the elements and keeping me warm and healthy. Warmth equals life.

The newly entered food data revealed my intake for a winterized menu was 2,153 calories. I adjusted the planner to include my heavier winter weight (around 132 to 133 pounds), and it *still* suggested 2,000 calories a day. According to *MyPyramid.gov* planner, I was now *over* my calorie limit and into the red area: the danger zone!

Figuring I was onto a major flaw in *MyPyramid.gov* recommendations and the way many people view dietary needs, I switched it up again. This time I entered the foods I would normally consume before and during my menstrual cycle. Oh the horror… my apologies to the manly men reading this. Physically, at my "special" time of the month, I crave more butter, fat, red meat, and food in general. My body needs the extra fat and cholesterol to create the hormones needed for a smooth flow and uses the protein to rebuild my uterine lining after it sheds. My hormone levels are in a constant state of flux throughout the month. Excess estrogen is required to build the uterine lining as it prepares the body for a potential pregnancy. If the egg is not fertilized, the uterine lining sheds and bleeding begins. It's as though menstruating women experience an internal surgery once per month. Before and after any surgery, it's imperative to give the body the foods (fuel) it needs to rebuild cells, recover energy, and create blood.

I believe that one of the many reasons women intensely crave chocolate, refined carbohydrates, and sugar (both before and during their period) is their bodies' way of *begging* for fat. Chocolate contains cocoa butter (fat), and sugar (which in excess turns to fat), and refined carbohydrates are another form of sugar that, if overeaten, turns to fat. Millions of women torment themselves with no-fat or low-fat diets thinking fat is bad and contributes to weight gain. The truth is eating little or *no* fat to achieve weight loss can be a dangerous and unhealthy practice. When your body's fat supply gets too low, it adversely affects not only the menstrual cycle, but the bones as well.[3] Loss of menstrual cycle, irregular menstrual cycle, and osteoporosis are all symptoms of inadequate body fat. When I feel the physical need for extra fat and/or protein, I give my body what it is asking for without judgment -- end of story. That includes a yummy grass-fed cheeseburger on a whole grain bun with a side of butter-sautéed vegetables and French fries. Yes, you read that correctly. Occasionally, I eat potatoes that have been deep fried and miraculously live to tell the tale! High temperature cooking, such as

---

3

http://www.betterhealth.vic.gov.au/bhcv2/bhcArticles.nsf/pages/Menstruat;ion_athletic_amenorrhoea?OpenDocument deep frying, roasting, and baking, is most likely to cause acrylamide formation. Acrylamide can cause nerve damage and cancer when eaten in large doses. It is found mainly in foods made from plants, such as potato products, grain products, or coffee.[4] French fries can contain these potentially dangerous substances so I do not eat them often (maybe once per month at most). Please keep in mind, it's not what we do once in a while that harms the human body… it's what we do on a daily basis.

After entering the amount of food I could consume on a premenstrual or menstrual day, I discovered my calorie intake was a whopping 2,581! Thank goodness I don't eat like that every day, but just when my body really needs it. It's clear my body's caloric needs change on a daily, monthly, and seasonal basis. In the winter, I eat 400 to 500 more calories than in the summer. And, when I get my period…. well… I can eat like a 300-pound linebacker! For the less sporty gals reading this, a linebacker is a *huge* football player (usually 6' 4" and 325 pounds) who protects the quarterback so he doesn't get squashed and flattened into a pancake. Make that a buckwheat pancake with grass-fed butter and real maple syrup, please.

Although the current USDA pyramid is a much more healthful version than its predecessor, it is still quite stagnant and biased. Every *body* is unique, and every person has his or her own individual dietary needs. I'll use Shaquille O'Neal as an extreme example. He's a popular basketball star who stands 7'1" and weighs 325 pounds; Shaq is a BIG man. I entered his information into the *MyPyramid.gov* website to see what the government thought would be a healthful amount of calories for

---

4

http://www.fda.gov/Food/FoodSafety/FoodContaminantsAdulteration/ChemicalContaminants/Acrylamide/ucm053569.htm him. The computer program redirected me to a page informing me "my weight is above the healthy range for my height," and recommended losing weight. Sorry Shaq... the government thinks you are fat.

Of course, Shaq is an extreme example of individual dietary needs. I'll relay one more not-so-extreme example of individuality, and then suggest how we can figure out our own bodily needs. My friend Donna is three inches taller than I, and weighs a little bit less (5'7" and 126 pounds). According to the USDA Pyramid planner, for her height, weight, and activity level she should be eating 2,200 calories per day. That means she *should* be able to eat *more* than I can. But she can't. And, it pisses her off! Even though I am physically smaller than she is, I have more muscle tone. She is softer and … shall I say… *squishier* (now she's really going to be pissed off!). My body burns calories at a quicker rate and I need to eat every 3 to 4 hours, whereas she can go 4 hours or more without refueling her system. She consumes far fewer calories than I do on any given day. If she were to eat the recommended 2,200 calories, she would surely be twice the woman she is now -- and, very, very angry!

All animals on earth know exactly what to eat and how much of it to put inside their bodies without resorting to an external calorie counter. There is also no Overeaters Anonymous or food recovery program for lions, tigers, and bears. Oh my! We need to take a lesson from the animal kingdom and learn how to eat.

Humans come in all shapes, sizes, and activity levels, and live in many different climates. All of these factors, and much more, dictate our food requirements. I commend the U.S. government for attempting to help us figure out how much and what to eat, but they don't take daily, monthly, or seasonal cycles into consideration. *You* need to do that. Some of the government recommendations at *MyPyramid.gov* are good: eat whole grains, a variety of vegetables, fruits, beans, meats, and good fats. It's imperative that you understand a few basic rules when creating a fully-balanced meal for your unique body:

- Every *body* has its own set of food requirements
- Do *not* adhere to a strict amount of calories
- Listen to bodily needs
- If you live in a temperate/seasonal climate, adjust your intake as your food requirements change with the weather
- Eat like a professional linebacker when necessary

With the above guidelines in mind, check out the government's nutritional information to help give you an understanding of how to create meals that *may* work for you, but remember to make personal adjustments. The pyramid's information is stagnant, but you are not. You are constantly changing from one day to the next.

The amount of food your body needs is entirely up to you. I realize this may put tremendous pressure on you, but you need to get back in touch with your physical body to become truly healthy. We habitually listen to other people telling us how much and what food to eat. But, how can other people possibly know your specific bodily needs? They don't live inside your body, and neither do I. Your body is yours and yours alone. Please own it. In time, you will discover you had the answers inside you; you just needed to get back in touch with that innate wisdom.

Deciphering our own physical needs may seem like a daunting task at first, but the more we do it, the easier it gets. Understanding food and our relationship to food are among our most intimate experiences. We physically take food into our bodies and it shapes us on a cellular level. We literally become that grilled cheese sandwich and French fries eaten at lunch. How does it feel? Good? Bad? Is this food relationship nourishing or exhausting? Is the food satisfying a physical or an emotional need? These are the questions you need to ask.

The categories of food are self-explanatory: whole grains and grain products, starchy vegetables, non-starchy vegetables, beans, animal proteins and animal products, fruits, fats, oils, nuts and seeds. These are all wholesome foods that humans have been eating for centuries; I will be elaborating on them in the following chapters.

Another vital piece of information to digest is that the foods in each category are *not* appropriate for everyone, no matter how healthful they may seem. Not all vegetables are good for all people, and that is also true of each of the other categories.

To broadly state that everyone should eat a specific food, I believe, is irresponsible. That's why it's imperative to get back to the basics and figure out what your unique body needs. As you read through this book, you will discover many types of foods you may want to taste. I advise you to try everything. Gauge how it feels inside you and pay attention to your body's physical, mental, and emotional reactions. It may or may not be the right food choice for you. Begin questioning how specific foods make you feel, no matter what you read in any book, including this one.

One way to unearth your body's innate wisdom is by keeping a food journal. As a teenager, I kept a journal to acknowledge my thoughts about life experiences. Jotting down thoughts helped connect me with my emotional self. It's the same thing with a food diary. Jot down notes indicating how your body feels physically, mentally, and emotionally after eating. This little bit of detective work can help you decipher what your body is saying, or in some cases, screaming! Below are some indicators that foods may not be working in your system:

- Gassiness and bloating
- Unusual sleepiness after meals
- Itchy eyes, ears, nose, or throat soon after eating
- Foods repeating on you
- Undigested or partially digested food in stool
- Emotional edginess after eating
- Fidgety or physically uncomfortable after eating or drinking
- Heart palpitations
- Sweet cravings between meals or after meals
- Headaches soon after eating
- Aches and pains
- Joints feeling sensitive or hot
- Excessive weight gain

These reactions, and many others, may indicate an undetected food allergy, weakened digestive system, organ system imbalance, or other dysfunction. The food and drinks we consume may or may not be working for us. In this day and age, we've come to ignore bodily reactions and continue ingesting substances that may not benefit us. It's time to reconnect to understand our bodies' messages.

Humans have a tendency to scientifically overthink food and its so-called healthful substances (fiber, phytonutrients, antioxidants, good fats, vitamins, and minerals). I was guilty of this behavior, too. Before I really began listening to my body, I bought into all the "healthy" gibberish and neglected what my body was trying to say to me. No matter what it says about the benefits of flax oil, I was unable to fully digest the stuff. I awoke every morning with swollen eye bags and excess mucus and congestion, until I restricted my intake, or cut flax oil out of my diet completely.

My clients are encouraged to keep a food diary, and within a few weeks many realize their bodies are talking to them with both subtle and not-so-subtle signs and clues. An older client complained of an inability to sleep through the night. She would wake two or three times to urinate and was exhausted from this interrupted sleep pattern. The doctor informed her that because of her age, her bladder was growing weaker. During her health consultation with me, she mentioned that during the day she suffered from frequent bouts of heart-racing anxiety. At the time, she was drinking 2 to 3 cups of coffee per day. I suggested she cut out caffeine for two weeks and see what would happen. Within one week, she noticed less anxiety and less nightly urination. By the time we spoke again two weeks later, she was no longer waking during the night at all. She also made the connection in her food diary that on the days she *did* consume coffee/caffeine, her heart raced uncomfortably. This is not rocket science. It's listening to the body and honoring it on a deeper level.

Another client consistently experienced headaches in the middle of her forehead that spread to the top of her head whenever she ate wheat bread, pasta, or anything containing wheat. She told me she was eating "whole wheat" because she read in a health magazine that it was good for her. I suggested she stop eating whole wheat products and switch to quinoa pasta, starchy vegetables, or gluten-free grains. Within a few days, the headaches ceased. It's possible she had an underlying wheat allergy, gluten intolerance, and/or overgrowth of Candida yeast.

A young client in her early twenties felt bloated and gassy after eating breakfast and lunch and couldn't figure out why. Her day began with dry hard breakfast cereal topped with soy milk, followed by soy yogurt and fruit for lunch. I informed her of the risks of eating *nonfermented* soy products. These dangers are discussed in the following chapter and in my previous book, ***The Whole Truth Eating and Recipe Guide***. We also discussed the hazards of eating highly processed hard breakfast cereals. There is more info on this topic in the "From Porridge to Prosperity" chapter in this book. Once the *nonfermented* soy and highly refined breakfast cereal were removed from her diet the bloating disappeared. Anytime she added them back in, the bloating returned.

An overweight client was consuming large amounts of raw salad daily because she thought it was good for her and would contribute to weight loss, a common mistake many dieters make. She complained of a *heavy* feeling in both her belly and legs soon after eating. Her food diary helped her discover that raw salads gave her an uncomfortable feeling, while cooked vegetables did not. The simple act of switching from eating mostly raw salads to more cooked vegetables easily helped her lose the excess weight - almost 10 pounds in one month! She still eats refreshing raw salads, but certainly not in the quantity she used to.

As for myself, I really enjoy the flavor of raw sweet red peppers, but they have a tendency to repeat on me, sometimes for hours. Accepting this information about the way my body works, I still enjoy peppers in small quantities, but will not eat them if I have to give a speech. Otherwise I would surely be burping my way through the seminar.

One more note on understanding the body. I recently attended a three-day chef's seminar in New York City. It was a seventy-two hour eating fest, sampling various cheeses and naturally cured meats from around the world; extra buttery butterfat, foie-gras, wild sustainable fish and game, and many other animal fats and proteins passed through my lips. I was hard-pressed to find a vegetable or piece of fruit among the display booths. By day two of the seminar, I noticed a slightly uncomfortable feeling on the right side of my body, inside my hip and below my rib cage. Intuitively, I thought my appendix and/or gallbladder were getting a tougher workout than they were used to. By day three, the pain on the right side of my body was strong and sharp. I knew I had to quit chewing the excess fat (literally) and get some fresh fruit and veggies into my system otherwise my appendix or gallbladder might burst!

I listened to my body's signals and began the third day with a light breakfast of simple rolled oats with walnuts, raisins, cinnamon, and a dollop of yogurt on top; a sweet ripe plum as midmorning snack; mesclun greens salad and a small amount of fish (about two or three ounces) for lunch; and a simple gazpacho soup with whole grain bread for dinner. The pain disappeared! Granted, the pain would've disappeared sooner had I fasted the entire day rather than eat, but when I don't eat, I get *grouchy*!

These are a handful of examples. As mentioned, every *body* is unique and what works for one person may not work for another. It's up to you to figure that out. Understanding the inner workings of your body will take time, so you'll need to be patient and loving as you get to know yourself on a deeper and more intimate level. It helps to have a solid support system or a professional health practitioner to work with to help figure out what your body is initially saying. I highly recommend working with a Holistic Health Counselor/Coach (like me!), a Traditional or Classical Chinese Medicine Practitioner, Intuitive Healer, Naturopathic Doctor, Food Coach, or anyone else you can trust and work with on a regular basis.

As far as the *quantity* of food to eat, I always suggest beginning with *less* than what your eyes tell you they want. When I was younger and didn't have the food sense I have now, I remember my mom looking at a plate of food that I had piled ten feet high and saying, "Ann, your eyes are bigger than your stomach." Later, she would find me splayed out on the couch with the top of my pants unbuttoned, hand gingerly rubbing my belly, suffering from a semiconscious food overdose. A good rule of thumb is to take less than you think you want; you can always return for seconds. Listening to the physical body is the most fundamental way to decipher how much to eat, and whether or not a specific food is right for your system.

I cannot finish this chapter without mentioning the emotional aspect of eating as well. It's imperative to listen to our emotional selves to help discover our needs. Many times, eating late at night, overeating, or eating when not hungry can indicate unresolved emotional issues such as loneliness, stress, fear, boredom, anxiety, anger, and others.

When I was initially building my business, I worked *all* the time. I would often find myself home alone at night working late, and feel compelled to rush out to the nearest health food store and purchase a big bag of chocolate-covered almonds or other sweet treats. I had no physical craving for that food. For me, it was purely comfort I was seeking. I desired sweets when feeling lonely and/or overworked. Today, when I'm feeling lonely, I reach out to family members or phone a friend. This connection fills me up in a way that chocolate-covered almonds never could. It fuels me with the love and companionship I was truly craving. Don't get me wrong, I still eat sweet treats occasionally, but not to shut off or downplay my emotions. Emotional eating is not healthful and it contributes to many diseases. Today, I allow myself to feel whatever I feel, and then find a healthful way to release or resolve those emotions.

Keeping a food diary helps us discover and disarm binge triggers. Are you angry at your boss or spouse? Are you scared? Lonely? Depressed? Anxious? Bored? Are old unresolved feelings coming up? We all have emotions, but many of us may not be conscious of our reaction to them. The tendency to push emotions aside, not feel them, or swallow them is very common. Just ask anyone suffering from an ulcer how often they swallow their emotions.

Write down whatever emotion is surfacing, then feel it, release it, and let it go. It may take thousands of pages of journaling before you find the answers that can help resolve some of these underlying issues. Don't worry… you've got your whole life to figure this stuff out. The answers may come in one week, one year, or one lifetime. It's imperative to be patient and loving with both your physical and emotional bodies as you move toward understanding yourself more intimately. Love and accept yourself as you go through the process of figuring out how best to invest in your physical and emotional needs. You can do it! I believe in you and your healing process.

As you can see from the wealth of information in this chapter, creating a fully balanced meal can include many aspects of food (physical, mental, spiritual, and emotional), and not just what we pile on our plate. Human beings are far more complex than a computer-generated calorie and fat counter.

I believe one of the best places to begin getting to know our needs is by performing the simple acts of self care and home cooking. The more we actively take part in the basics of cooking and caring for ourselves, the deeper our knowledge of food and how it affects us can become. The following chapter reveals how, why, and where to purchase the best quality foods so you can begin the process of investing in your health.... one meal at a time!

Chapter 3

PUT YOUR MONEY WHERE YOUR MOUTH IS!

It's time to stock up the pantry (and your body) with the best food money can buy. Many health conscious consumers read labels to help guide their purchases. Unfortunately, packaging labels and many of their listed ingredients can be deceptive and misleading. Ugh! Where the heck are the USDA watchdogs when we need them? It's time to get to know what the labels *really* mean so we can begin investing our money in the best quality foods.

ORGANIC

According to the USDA, "100% Organic" means the final product is free from synthetic fertilizers, pesticides, genetically modified organisms, irradiation, antibiotics, and hormones. This is important -- especially if you want food that's free from synthetic chemicals and other carcinogenic crap! Going organic is a smart choice. But... there's a little snafu in the government's "organic" labeling process, and it affects small local farmers and subsequently you, the consumer.

"Producers who market less than $5000 worth of organic products are not required to become certified but must still adhere to the federal standards for organic production, product labeling and handling, including keeping appropriate records, and [they] *cannot* use the USDA seal."[5]

---

[5] http://asap.sustainability.uiuc.edu/org-ag/org-cert/

That basically means that small local farmers, even though they may be growing things *organically,* cannot legally use the "USDA Certified Organic" label. Why is it that anytime the government gets involved, the little guys get screwed?

Let's start a food revolution and purchase most, if not all, of our products from small local farmers. To join this culinary crusade, all you need to do is purchase food from your local farmers market. That's it. There is no need to storm the streets protesting loudly with bullhorns or dump tea into the harbor. Purchase from the little guys (and gals) who need our financial support to keep producing great quality food without having to pay HUGE fees for a label they cannot afford. Remember to *ask* the farmer how the produce or livestock is raised -- even though it may *not* be labeled as such, it may still be organic and/or naturally grown.

There is a grass-roots movement happening across America that both supports the local farmers who can't get USDA certified and ensures that products are grown with the highest principles and ideals. This organization holds to standards for organic that go above and beyond those of the USDA. Look for the Certified Naturally Grown (CNG) label or check out their website for more information.[6]

NATURAL

The "natural" label has been horribly abused and can be used on practically any product to market *anything*. "Natural" products can contain chemicals, pesticides, synthetic hormones, genetically modified organisms... you name it. Essentially, "Natural" products may not be natural at all.

---

[6] http://www.naturallygrown.org/

FREE RANGE/FREE ROAMING

Eggs and poultry can be labeled "free-range" or "free-roaming" if the animals have access to the outdoors. This does *not* mean they actually make it to the outside world. "Access to the outdoors" could mean there is a small window or entryway the size of Alice in Wonderland's tiny little door, but that the animals never go through it to experience a life filled with barnyard adventures. Can you imagine what it would feel like to live inside without access to the outdoors your entire life? There is no doubt that your bones would be frail from lack of vitamin D, sunshine, exercise, and your immune system would be terribly weak. The same thing happens to animals that are not allowed outside to roam freely. It's important to make sure your poultry *really* is "free-range" or "free roaming." The best and surest way to discover this information is to actually visit a local farm and see how the farmer is raising the animals. If visiting a farm is not an option, then you have to let go and trust that the integrity of the product is true.

PASTURE-RAISED or PASTURED

"Pastured" means the animals have been raised on a pasture (outdoors) where they are free to roam and eat seeds, grass, bugs, worms, and all other delicious things they are designed to eat. These animals have access to fresh air, sunshine, exercise and many other aspects of nature. Pastured animals live a better quality life and can therefore supply us with more healthful and tastier meats and dairy products.

GRASS-FED

I understand this may seem like an odd concept, but "grass-fed" literally means the animal has been fed grass, which for them is an ideal diet. Cows and other ruminants are physically designed to digest grass –

ingesting anything else (for example corn and soy) makes them sick. This is one of the many reasons our livestock are fed a steady diet of antibiotics – to help keep them alive. “Grass-fed” is on the top of my list when searching for meat products. However, a "grass-fed" label doesn't mean the animal was fed grass its entire life. Some grass-fed cattle are "grain-finished." That means they were fed grains to fatten them up prior to slaughter. Some people prefer grain-finished animals because they are fattier. I prefer grass-fed animals. They are leaner and tend to be healthier overall. The healthier the animal is, the healthier you will be when you eat it.

There are so many labels on food products in the market -- healthful, heritage, fair trade, fresh, good source, fat-free, calorie-free, GMO- free -- that it can make your head spin! Be wary of food labels and read ingredients carefully. The best way to know what is in your food is to either grow it yourself (even I’m not that idealistic…yet!) or get to know your local farmers and ask them how they are growing their products.

Organic, local, seasonal, and pasture raised foods are some of the best products money can buy. These are foods that have sustained human health for centuries, long before chemicals, pesticides, additives, preservatives, advertising, marketing, and fancy packaging entered the marketplace and mucked everything up. Some of these better quality foods may cost a bit more, but I’ll show you how to offset that cost in the coming chapters so you will get more food for your money! Always remember that buying better quality food is an investment in your health, and you’re worth it. If we can spend big bucks on expensive clothes to beautify the outside of our bodies, we can spend a little extra money purchasing foods that will beautify the inside of the body as well. Not only that, but we don't even think twice about having three televisions, two cars, computers, ipods, and other expensive gadgets; but when it comes to our food, we hesitate to spend that money. I believe we need to reevaluate where to spend our money so it can benefit our life the most.

The newest food trend on the market, "locavore," advises us to purchase and eat what grows in our immediate environment. This is a fantastic concept, but it's certainly not a new one. Humans have traditionally eaten locally grown seasonal foods. Modern technology has changed our traditional way of eating; and today, every type of food is available at any time of the year regardless of the season or environment in which it is grown. This may sound like an amazing leap for mankind, but it's not. Our modern way of eating *everything from everywhere* not only destroys the environment by burning large amounts of fossil fuel to ship foods to and from faraway places, it also weakens the digestive system, contributes to yeast overgrowth, and poor calcium absorption. According to Dr. John Matsen, ND, the more sun that plants are exposed to, the more potassium and sugar they produce. High potassium and sugar levels alert your kidneys that you're out in the hot sun and that your skin must be making vitamin D. Therefore, if you eat foods from hot sunny climates during the cold wintry months, your kidneys don't activate stored vitamin D, inhibiting absorption of calcium.[7]

Another perspective from Traditional Chinese Medicine reveals that salads, vegetables, and fruits are *cooling* to the body. During the hot summer months, this cooling effect can be quite beneficial for most people; but during the cold winter season, it creates a damp spleen

[7] Eating Alive II, Dr. John Matsen N.D., Goodwin Books, Ltd, 2004, pp. 23-27

condition, gas, bloating, cold hands and feet, and eventually leads to other more serious ailments.

Eating locally and seasonally grown food aligns our internal environment (the body and its organs) with the external environment (the view outside our window) creating a body that is physically stronger and prepared for the elements. For example, on a steamy hot summer day, I would probably choose crisp salad greens, juicy watery fruits, freshly caught fish, and other cooling foods that are abundantly available at that time of year; they would cool my body so I can better handle the heat. On the other hand, if I look outside my window and there is a thick blanket of icy snow covering the ground, and people are trudging through the streets bundled up in winter snorkel jackets, my innate wisdom tells me that *cooling* summer foods would make my body work twice as hard to heat up. More appropriate food for a cold snowy day might be a hearty stew made with bone stock, grass-fed meat, beans, and root vegetables, and a honkin' hunk of warm sourdough bread slathered with pastured butter.

When you invest in locally harvested food, it can enhance immunity and reduce and/or eliminate allergies entirely. For example, eating honey from bees living in or near your immediate environment can be more beneficial than taking allergy shots and medication. The bees travel from flowers to plants, to trees, and back to the hive carrying a variety of pollens on their fuzzy little bodies. Eating honey with these trace amount of pollens can build immunity, naturally. After all, an allergy shot is an injection of the very substance we are allergic to. If you are sick and tired of spending spring, summer, and fall sneezing your head off and scratching your itchy eyeballs out of their red-rimmed sockets, eating locally grown foods can help you find relief. This includes eating all local foods: vegetables and fruits, poultry, eggs, meat, and butter from grass-fed or pastured animals.

It's easy to discover what's growing in your environment by checking out the local farmers market. A traditional farmer cannot grow something incompatible with his environment. Locate sustainable food, Community Supported Agriculture, butchers, bakers, restaurants, chefs, and farmers markets near you by going to Eatwellguide.org, Localharvest.org, or Sustainabletable.org and enter your zip code. It's that easy. There is also a "Resources" page at the back of this book, and a video blog on my website that showcases where to find great quality food. Go to www.AndreaBeaman.com, and watch the videos to find food, fabulous food, all over the country!

If you do *not* have the desire or time to hunt for food at the farmers market, good quality products can be purchased at any Whole Foods, Trader Joe's, Wild By Nature, gourmet market, or local health food store. The following chapter can help you navigate our compromised food supply within the aisles of a supermarket.

Chapter 4

THIS LITTLE PIGGY WENT TO THE MARKET

Some people cringe at the thought of venturing into a health food market– it scares the dickens out of them! They think the food tastes bad, or it's too complicated to make, or somehow they are going to be inducted into a cult of alfalfa-sprout-eating, wheat-grass-drinking hippies. "Peace, man, peace. Please pass the herbs."

Thanks to the growing demand for better quality foods, many mainstream supermarkets carry organically grown local foods and pasture raised animal products. Better food choices are available because people are getting hip (like those happy hippies!) and have made the connection that our food directly affects our health. "You are what you eat." If we consistently eat better food, we ensure a more productive and healthful life.

THE LIST

For many folks, food shopping can be overwhelming, so it's imperative to arrive at the market prepared. Bring a written list of items and, even more importantly, venture into the marketplace only on a full stomach. Shopping on an empty stomach could be catastrophic to health. Supermarkets are huge warehouses stocked with mountains of food. Our survival instincts kick into high gear when we are famished and stumble upon all that food, glorious food! We have a tendency to grab anything off the shelf, no matter what it is, even if we have no desire for it. I'm sure this has happened to you at one time or another – you come home from the grocery store with items you had not intended to buy, and wonder, "How the heck did these low-fat cookies, baked potato chips, and fat-free frozen yogurt pops get in here?" It would be nice to think that somehow those foods leapt off the shelves, or forcibly jumped out of the freezer and into your cart. I could title that chapter, "When Junk Food Attacks!" We will always reach for foods that may not benefit us if our bodies are in starvation mode.

Shopping with a fully satisfied belly and a written list keeps us focused on what is absolutely *needed.* You'll be better equipped to get in and out of the market with minimal or no damage to your hips, waist, buttocks, and bank account. To help guide you toward wise food choices, I've included a simple shopping list at the end of this chapter.

PURCHASE PRODUCE

At the market, my first stop is always the produce section, no matter what season it is. There are many vegetables that are staples in my kitchen because they are available year-round. Always remember that what goes into your shopping basket will eventually become part of your body, so fill that basket wisely. Grab a bunch of dark leafy greens like kale, collard greens, arugula, or bok choy. While you're at it, throw in some cancer-fighting cruciferous vegetables (also known as the brassicacae family of vegetables) like broccoli and cauliflower. Then add carrots, cabbage, parsley, and squashes, too. And last, but certainly not least, toss in some members of the allicacae family: onions, garlic, scallions, shallots,. leeks, and chives. These are the perennial bulbous plants that produce chemical compounds which give them the characteristic onion or garlic taste and odor[8] and have been traditionally used to promote warmth, resolve blood stagnancies, and reduce clotting. They are rich in sulfur and have an antifungal and antimicrobial effect in the body that helps to eliminate unfavorable yeast and bacteria.[9] And, no body likes unfavorable bacteria. Gross!

Vegetables contain chlorophyll, calcium, iron, folic acid, fiber, antioxidants, and many other nutrients. But, I don't want you to focus on the *micronutrients* in these foods. I want you to focus on the *wholeness* of food. Once we spotlight and extract specific beneficial nutrients inside food instead of eating the actual food itself in its entirety, it loses its healthful value in many ways. "…as soon as you remove these useful molecules from the context of the whole foods they're found in, as we've done in creating antioxidant supplements, they don't work at all. Indeed, in the case of beta carotene ingested as a supplement, scientists have discovered that it actually increases the risk of certain cancers."[10]

Scientific studies have revealed shocking information about vitamin and mineral supplements. According to the Journal of the American Medical Association, antioxidant vitamins increased a person's risk of dying by up to 16%! The University of Washington found that vitamin E elevated lung cancer risk, and researchers at the National Cancer Institute found that men who took more than one multivitamin daily had higher rates of prostate cancer.[11] Holy guacamoles! These are scary statistics.

---

[8] http://en.wikipedia.org/wiki/Allium
[9] Healing With Whole Foods, Paul Pitchford, North Atlantic books 1993, p505
[10] www.nytimes.com/2007/01/28/magazine/28nutritionism.t.html?pagewanted=4&_r=2 – Michael Pollan
[11] http://www.rd.com/living-healthy/are-vitamins-really-that-good-for-you-/article46647.html

Animals in the wild do not need supplements to thrive and neither do humans. Wholesome food contains all the elements we need in perfect balance: fiber, water, protein, fat, vitamins, minerals, carbohydrates, and antioxidants. We are a part of nature; our bodies will use what they need from our food and naturally discard the waste. Overdoses of isolated supplements accumulate in the body and wreak havoc on our finely tuned system. In the short term, supplements may do some good, but in thc long term, they can cause serious damage.

Keep in mind that there are better and more delicious ways to get the vitamins and minerals your body needs without toxic side effects. Get into the habit of purchasing "whole" foods with all of their nutrients intact. We cannot create better long-term health and wellness by eating isolated nutrients.

After filling your basket with a bevy of beautiful vegetables, venture into the fruit section. Fruit can help satisfy sweet cravings. Grab a couple of crisp apples, succulent pears, juicy plums, plump peaches, or a box of fresh berries. As mentioned in the previous chapter, choose fruit and vegetables that are local and in season because they will be the best food for your body, and they will taste better. The concept of seasonal and local eating is used at many great restaurants around the world. Smart chefs understand that when food is in season it always tastes the freshest, the ripest, and the best. People pay top dollar to sit in some of the finest restaurants because they know they're getting a magnificent meal. The food we purchase is a delicious investment, and our return on our investment can be felt and seen in the health of our bodies.

WHOLESOME GOODNESS

There seems to be a lot of confusion around whole grains, and good and bad carbohydrates. I think the pandemonium occurred somewhere along the path of human food consumption when someone erroneously stated that *all* carbohydrates were bad. Who knows how it happened? I can only guess that maybe an innocent victim was wolfing down an oversized bagel too quickly and it got lodged in his throat. He dropped dead on the spot with the bagel hanging suspiciously out of his mouth. A bystander witnessing this tragedy shouted, "Look! Carbohydrates kill!" And thus carbo-phobia was born and *all* carbs were labeled bad.

Once we become educated about the effects of "good and "bad" carbohydrates in the human body, irrational fears will subside and bread makers around the world can fire up their ovens again and get back to work! Some of the "good" carbohydrates to stock in your home are whole grains and whole grain products. Whole grains have been part of the human food supply for thousands of years, and recipes for them have been passed down from generation to generation. There is even a reference to whole grains and bread making in the Bible. "Take thou also unto thee wheat, and barley, and beans, and lentils, and millet, and spelt, and put them in one vessel, and make thee bread thereof; according to the number of the days that thou shalt lie upon thy side, even three hundred and ninety days, shalt thou eat thereof.[12] Yes, that's right… the Bible is actually a big old cookbook. Dust it off, say a prayer, and start cooking. Amen, sister!

---

[12] http://bible.cc/ezekiel/4-9.htm

Whole grains are wholesome foods that haven't been completely refined. They are "whole" as the name implies, have not been broken down; they retain their integrity. They contain most of their vitamins, minerals, bran, fiber, protein, carbohydrates, and other essential elements that make them a better food choice than most refined grain products like white flour, white pasta, white rice and the infamous white killer bagel!

A good rule of thumb: the whiter the grain, the more anemic it may be. It's clearly a wise idea to go for the *brown* when making carbohydrate choices. This does not mean that chocolate cake, although quite brown, should be considered a good carbohydrate choice.

A simple example of whole and refined grains is brown rice versus white rice. These are actually the same grain, only the white rice has been stripped of its outer layers (bran, fiber, nutrients, and vitamins), leaving behind a refined carbohydrate with a high glycemic index. Foods with a high glycemic index turn to sugar rapidly in the body, and, when eaten in excess, create blood sugar swings and nutritional deficiencies. You could probably eat five bowls of white rice and become quite full, but the body's nutritional needs may not be met, so you might still be hungry for nutrients.

I know what you're thinking… and yes, you can still eat white rice, white flour, and white killer bagels; just keep in mind that the greatest health potential can be reached if you consume whole grains and whole grain products *most* often, and highly refined grains (and chocolate cake) *less* often. Learning how to get healthy should never be about deprivation. "Preserving the health by too strict a regimen is a wearisome malady." François Duc de la Rochefoucauld.

At the market, pick up a bag of brown rice, barley, wild rice, quinoa, polenta, kasha, millet, or whole, rolled, or cracked oats. As long as the bags are sealed tightly, they can be kept in the cabinet.

When I first began buying whole grains, I would occasionally discover small moths in my pantry and wonder, "Where the heck are these furry little flying creatures coming from?" It's not as if I had a sweater hanging amongst the canned goods and tomato sauce. I discovered the bugs were coming from the opened bags of grains. Oh, the horror! It completely turned me off from eating these wholesome foods. After my shock subsided, I realized the bugs were there because there were no preservatives or chemicals on the grains. It was a nourishing food to eat and even the bugs knew it. And, for those of you who are totally grossed out about the "bug factor," keep in mind that the U.S. government (FDA) allows a certain amount of animal feces, bug bodies, rodent hair, and other unsavory elements into prepackaged foods. At least, if you buy whole grains and other whole foods, you have the option of picking these things out and discarding them from your meal. When buying packaged and ready-made foods, you lose that option because the "unsavory bug ingredients" are already incorporated into the food. Bleacch!

The way to eliminate any potential bug problems is to make sure grains are sealed tightly in glass jars or kept in the refrigerator. This will help maintain freshness and extend shelf life, too. Don't bug out, just keep the bugs out.

Other grain products to purchase are pastas and noodles. There are many varieties: udon, soba, somen, and rice noodles, or quinoa, corn, spelt, kamut, rice, whole wheat, and durum semolina pastas. Although pastas are refined grains, they have been nourishing healthy people for centuries (most notably the Asians and Italians!). And, pasta is a great staple to have on hand because it's quick and easy to prepare.

Whole grain breakfast cereals are another great choice. They have been partially refined and cracked and usually are quick cooking, too. Some examples include rolled oats, multigrain porridge, cream of wheat, cream of buckwheat (one of my favorites), cream of rye, and many more. The "cream of" on the package doesn't mean there is cream in it. These cereals become creamy when you simply cook them in water; but you can also use whole milk or cream, almond milk, oat milk, or other milk. Make sure the package says whole grain or cracked grain and nothing else.

Hearty grain breads, wraps, and tortillas are good carbohydrate choices and are quite wholesome, nutritious, and delicious. One of the reasons most bread has been shelved with a bum rap is that many are highly refined, nutritionally deficient, white flour products, and are not good for health. Even some of the heavily marketed, "whole grain breads," are actually highly refined white flour products with vitamins, minerals, and coloring *added* to make them look more healthful than they are. Looks can be deceiving! If the ingredient list is quite long and you cannot pronounce the words, it's probably not a wise choice. The ingredient list should be simple with words a second grader could pronounce. If it's unpronounceable, it's probably indigestible. Better quality bread may have listed as ingredients whole wheat, whole grains, water, yeast, and sea salt. With nutritious bread as a staple in your home, you'll be able to make quick lunches and simple sandwiches and snacks when there is no time to cook.

BOUNTIFUL BEANS

Dried beans are usually kept in the same aisle as the whole grains, so you don't have to go very far for your next items. Beans are a great source of fiber, potassium, calcium, iron, B vitamins, and other health-promoting nutrients. If you're feeling inspired, and have time to cook, purchase dried beans: black beans (turtle beans), black-eyed peas, garbanzos (chick-peas), northern beans, navy beans, kidney beans, lentils (red, green, black, or brown), lima, anasazi, pinto, or any others. Store dried beans in glass jars or any airtight container to extend their shelf life for up to one year.

CAN IT!

I am not a big fan of canned foods. I definitely prefer fresh, local, and seasonal ingredients. But, sometimes there are days when I'm too darn tired or busy to cook! On those days, canned foods come in handy. One of the main caveats of eating canned foods is the high levels of toxic Bisphenol A (BPA) that has been linked with cancer and infertility.[13] BPA is the hard plastic coating used on the inside of canned food. For the sake of good health, eat fresh food most often and canned food least often.

If you cannot allot time in your schedule to cook beans from scratch, canned beans can be an alternative. As with all canned products, purchase cans free of dents, cracks, and bulging lids which could mean that the safety of the food has been compromised. Canned beans can safely be stored in your pantry for 2 to 5 years.[14] Also, be conscious of

---

[13] http://www.ewg.org/reports/bisphenola%20

[14] http://hgic.clemson.edu/factsheets/HGIC3520.htm

the salt content and seek out brands made with sea salt (a better quality salt) or Kombu (sea vegetable). Remember to rinse canned beans before eating them to help release some of their gaseous properties.

Some other canned foods to purchase are canned fish like wild salmon, sardines, anchovies, kippers, and tuna – whichever you enjoy most. A healthful hint about canned sardines and salmon: if you are seeking an extra boost of calcium purchase them with bones intact rather than the skinless boneless type. Bones are a great source of calcium; and once the sardine or salmon is mashed to make a delicious salad, the bones break down and you don't even know they are there. Remember, if you acquire your calcium and essential fats in the food they naturally come with, your body will have an easier time digesting and absorbing the nutrients. I've had many clients who complained they could not digest fish oil pills (The oil kept repeating on them or gave them a stomach ache). Once they stopped eating the fish oil pills and started eating the actual fish in its whole flesh form with all of the other nutrients intact, the indigestion magically disappeared. Voila!

Tuna (both fresh and canned), because of its high mercury content, is best not eaten too often, maybe one or two times per month. And, if you are pregnant, you should steer clear of tuna and other large predatory fish (shark, king mackerel, tile fish, grouper, and swordfish) entirely – mercury is not healthful for the fetus and it contributes to birth defects, severe damage to the nervous system, brain damage, learning disabilities, and hearing loss.[15] [16]

[15] http://www.americanpregnancy.org/pregnancyhealth/fishmercury.htm
[16] http://www.marchofdimes.com/pnhec/159_15759.asp

Other canned items to stock in the pantry include diced tomatoes, stewed tomatoes, and tomato paste. Canned tomatoes and other high-acid foods such as juices, fruits, pickles, and sauerkraut can keep in the pantry for 12 to 18 months. Low acid foods such as vegetables and meat can be stored for two years or longer.

BOTTLES AND BUTTERS

Now, let's get some *natural* peanut butter, almond butter, sesame tahini, and other spreadable goodies. Make sure these products are made from nuts and seeds, maybe a little sea salt, and **nothing else**. Most commercial (popular) brands of nut butter contain hydrogenated oils and added sugars. These are the ingredients we want to eliminate from our diet. Better quality nut butters contain natural oils (essential fatty acids and vitamin E) that usually separate and rise to the top of the jar. If you mix the contents of the jar thoroughly and put the nut butters inside the refrigerator, the oil will not separate.

Pick up natural fruit jams to complement those nut butters. Choose brands that are sweetened only with fruit and fruit juice. Fruits contain enough sugar in the form of fructose that jams and jellies don't need added sugar to make them sweet. At least make an effort to buy brands that don't have sugar listed as the first ingredient. A good thing to remember about ingredient labels is that the ingredient that the product contains most of is listed first. Choosing better quality nut butters and jams makes it easy for you to create quick and easy sandwiches for you and the kiddies. C'mon… who doesn't like munching on a PB&J every once in a while? For those of you who don't know what a PB&J is, it's a peanut butter and jelly sandwich. And, if you've never had one, you may be missing out on one of the most simple and fun snacks foods ever created. It is literally fat (nut butter) and sugar (fruit) on bread (oh the horror!), and it is yummy!

SUPPORTIVE SNACKS

Purchase raw or dry-roasted nuts and seeds for snacks or to sprinkle on salads, grains, and other foods. Nuts and seeds contain essential fatty acids, vitamin E, and other vitamins and minerals that can benefit health. For the best quality and freshest choices, buy nuts in air-tight packages or still inside their shells. Varieties of nuts and seeds include walnuts, almonds, pecans, filberts, peanuts, pine nuts, pistachios, sesame seeds, pumpkin seeds, and sunflower seeds. Nuts and seeds contain fats so you only need a small amount, chewed well, to reap their nutritional benefits. Eaten in large quantities, oily nuts and seeds can contribute to sluggish digestion (gas and bloating), but one or two handfuls per day can be a highly energizing snack.

CONTRIBUTING CONDIMENTS & OTHER GOOD STUFF

Purchase condiments like mustard and ketchup but check the labels to make sure there isn't any high fructose corn syrup listed as an ingredient. I keep prepared mustard in the house to make dressings and sauces. Earl Mindell and Virginia Hopkins, authors of "Prescription Alternatives," blame our nation's sharp rise in diabetes on increased consumption of high fructose corn syrup and the resulting depletion of chromium in the body. Mindell and Hopkins say that studies done at the U.S. Department of Agriculture's Human Nutrition Resource Center reveal that consuming fructose in this form causes chromium levels to drop, in turn raising LDL cholesterol and triglyceride levels and impairing immune system function. "As our consumption of high fructose corn syrup has risen 250 percent in the past 15 years, our rate of diabetes has increased approximately 45 percent in about the same time period," said Mindell.[17] High fructose corn syrup is a cheap sweetener added to almost everything on supermarket shelves. Steer clear of this disease-promoting ingredient, and opt for natural sweeteners that have been around for thousands of years. Our ancestors weren't riddled with diabetes, heart disease, cancer, or many other ailments that have been linked to this dangerous and cheap sugar permeating our food supply. Pick up real maple syrup, raw honey, granulated cane juice, or beet sugar, and remember to use these sweeteners in moderation. Don't overdo it. After all… they are still forms of sugar, and sugar is not the best source for wholesome nutrition.

Cold-pressed vegetable oils will make your food taste savory and delicious. For light cooking and flavoring foods, choose good quality extra virgin olive and regular olive oils, sesame and toasted sesame oils, peanut oil, and walnut oil. For higher-heat cooking, saturated fats like coconut oil and animal fats (chicken fat, duck fat, lard, beef tallow) are best. They don't oxidize or turn rancid as quickly as polyunsaturated and monounsaturated fats.

Vinegars are another great addition to your pantry. There are so many flavored vinegars on the market that it's hard to keep track of them all. Let's stick with the basics for now: balsamic, apple cider, rice, red and white wine, and champagne vinegars. These are all good choices.

I also like to keep jars of Kalamata olives and capers in my cupboard. Hey, ya never know who's coming over for dinner. And, with the addition of a couple of capers or olives, you can change the flavor and appeal of a boring pasta sauce into something more fancy-schmancy!

---

[17] http://www.newstarget.com/009333.html

SASSY SEASONINGS

One of the biggest mistakes I find people making when they begin eating better is the tendency to eat boring, flavorless food. They think in order for the dish to be "healthful," it should also be bland. To prevent this tasteless disaster from happening in your kitchen, jazz up your meals with fresh herbs and dried seasonings. Besides making food tastier and more exciting, they actually enhance digestion by stimulating our senses and promoting the production of digestive juices. Unrefined noniodized sea salt, peppercorns, and fresh or dried herbs like basil, bay leaves, dill, sage, thyme, and oregano are good choices. Spices like cinnamon, chili powder, cumin, coriander, curry, cayenne pepper can help jazz up meals. Spices, both whole and ground, do have a shelf life. Over time, spices lose potency and flavor, and then you are right back where you started eating lackluster food. Ideally, purchase spices whole and grind them yourself to extend their shelf life. If they have not been cracked or ground (exposing them to the air), they can last up to four years in an airtight container. If you don't have the time or desire to buy and grind your own whole spices, you can buy ground spices, which have a shorter shelf life, usually between two and three years. Spices should be stored in a cool, dry place and not directly above the stove. Whole or ground spices that have lost their aroma are too old to use. Dried herbs keep for less time than dried spices. Most herbs last between one and two years. You can test herbs by crushing them lightly in between your fingers or in the palm of your hand. If the herbs smell flavorful, they are still good. If they have no odor after crushing, toss them into the trash. Since dried herbs and spices keep for such long periods of time, consider them as a long-term investment in creating flavorful food.

It's also a good idea to store some type of bouillon cubes (vegetable, chicken, or beef), or containers of natural beef, chicken, or veggie stock. We'll be using stocks in upcoming chapters; I will teach you how to make them from scratch. If you want to try a recipe and don't have any of this homemade goodness stored in the freezer, the store-bought bouillon cubes and commercially prepared containers of stock can suffice.

TEATIME

If you want to kick the coffee habit to improve health and energy levels, grab a box of assorted green tea, black tea, or a variety of herbal teas like chamomile, licorice, peppermint, orange spice, passion fruit, rooibos, cranberry, or raspberry. There is such a wide variety of tea to choose from that most health food stores have entire aisles dedicated to tea. In many countries around the world, tea has long been associated with longevity and good health. It is the second most widely consumed beverage in the world, exceeded only by water. You can try a new flavor every week for a year and still have not experienced all the different types and combination of teas available on the market. If you happen to have a friend named Alice (or any other friend, for that matter), invite her over for a little tea party. It could be the beginning of an exciting tea-tasting adventure.

PURCHASING PERISHABLES

It's time to find the perishable items in the store's refrigerated section. Browse the meat counter and ask specifically for pasture fed, grass fed, or organic and naturally raised meats. "Grass fed products are rich in all the fats now proven to be health enhancing, but are low in the fats that have been linked with disease."[18] Purchase beef, buffalo, chicken, lamb, turkey, duck, pork, pheasant, and other wild game – whatever you prefer eating. Then swim over to the fish counter and purchase wild or locally caught fish. I find it's more time efficient and financially beneficial to buy meats, poultry, and fish in large or whole portions -- the entire animal when possible. (I will discuss the financial and healthful benefits of purchasing whole animals in a later chapter.) Then separate it into smaller pieces and store them in the freezer. If properly packaged in airtight moisture-proof bags or wraps, specifically intended for the freezer, frozen foods can be stored for 3 to 4 months at a time.

Next, travel to the dairy case, but steer clear of the margarine and butter substitutes that contain hydrogenated oils. These fats contribute to coronary heart disease and overall poor health.[19] Pick up real butter made from organic or pastured (grass fed) cows. "Butter contains lecithin, a substance that assists in the proper assimilation and metabolism of cholesterol and other fat constituents. Butter also contains a number of antioxidants that protect against the kind of free radical damage that weakens the arteries. Vitamin A and vitamin E found in butter both play a strong antioxidant role. Butter is a very rich source of selenium -- a vital antioxidant -- containing more per gram than herring or wheat germ."[20] Bottom line: butter is better! And, while at the dairy case, you can purchase full-fat natural yogurt or kefir with no added sweeteners. Fat helps our bodies absorb calcium and keeps us

[18] http://www.mercola.com/beef/health_benefits.htm
[19] http://news.bbc.co.uk/1/hi/health/3167764.stm
[20] http://www.westonaprice.org/foodfeatures/butter.html

feeling more satisfied physically. If you opt to eat any type of food without the fat, it naturally comes with, your body will search for that fat all day; and you may get wild cravings. Trust me, eat full-fat food -- just eat it in smaller quantities. For example, when I purchase a small container of full-fat yogurt, it lasts me three servings. I don't slurp down an entire container in one sitting, even if the package claims it's one serving. Do not listen to advice from the manufacturer of *any* product. Their job is to sell more products; the more you eat, the more they sell.

While in the dairy section, purchase free-roaming, naturally raised, or pastured eggs. Get a dozen. Contrary to popular belief, the egg, with its cholesterol rich yolk, is a very healthful food. Also, look for raw, unpasteurized sauerkraut and pickles. These are usually kept in the refrigerated section, too. These traditional foods are a wise purchase as they contain beneficial bacteria that can enhance digestion.

If you're feeling curious about trying new foods, pick up a container of tofu, tempeh, or miso from the refrigerated section of the store. These are traditionally prepared soy products that are beneficial to health. Soy has been touted as a "healthful" food, but it has to be properly processed for us to be able to access its nutritional benefits. Soybeans contain large amounts of phytic acid and trypsin inhibitors that block nutrient absorption. Traditional cultures, most notably the Asians, who ate soybeans, fermented them to release these anti-nutrients and make them digestible. In America, we've bypassed the fermentation process to quickly mass produce soybeans and have created some not-so-healthful products. Soy dogs, soy burgers, soy chips, soy nuts, soy oil, soy yogurt, isolated soy proteins, soy margarine, soy meats, and other nonfermented soy products can detrimentally affect health. Soy phytoestrogens disrupt endocrine function and have the potential to cause infertility and to promote breast cancer in adult women, and are potent antithyroid agents that cause hypothyroidism and may cause thyroid cancer. In infants, consumption of soy formula has been linked to autoimmune thyroid disease.[21] Choose soy products wisely. The soy products used in some of the recipes in this book are all wise choices.

Speaking of foods with an Asian flair, you could pick up some dried sea vegetables (seaweed) before you head out of the store. Sea vegetables offer the widest range of minerals that are found in the ocean – similar to the mineral content in human blood. This is a highly nutritious food for us. I know the thought of seaweed may scare some folks… have no fear. I can show you how to make them taste absolutely delicious.

Peruse the shopping list on the following pages, and get your beautiful body moving to the nearest store. You don't need to buy everything on the list, but do try to purchase something from each category. Begin stocking your home with the best quality food so we can get started with the cooking already. Yeah baby!

And, remember, when it comes to investing in your health… YOU ARE WORTH IT! "Gold that buys health can never be ill spent." Thomas Dekker, Westward Ho, 1604.

---

[21] http://www.westonaprice.org/component/content/section/6.html

Shopping List

Seasonal Vegetables	**Seasonal Fruit**	**Beans**
Arugula	Apples	Aduki
Bok Choy	Apricots	Anasazi
Broccoli	Berries	Black Turtle
Brussels Sprouts	Cherries	Cannellini
Butternut Squash	Cranberries	Garbanzo
Cabbage (red & green)	Grapes	Kidney
Carrots	Lemons	Lentils
Cauliflower	Melons	Navy
Chinese Cabbage	Peaches	Pinto
Collard Greens	Pears	Tofu
Cucumbers	Plums	
Daikon	Raisins	**Sea Vegetables**
Garlic	Watermelon	Arame
Ginger		Kelp
Kale	**Whole Grains**	Kombu
Leeks	Barley	Hiziki
Lettuces	Brown Rice	Nori
Mushrooms	Kasha	Wakame
Mustard Greens	Millet	
Onions	Oats	**Seeds and Nuts**
Parsley	Polenta	Almonds
Parsnips	Quinoa	Peanuts
Pumpkins		Pine Nuts
Radishes	**Whole Grain Bread**	Pumpkin Seeds
Rutabagas	Multigrain	Sesame Seeds
Savoy Cabbages	Rye	Sunflower Seeds
Scallions	Sourdough	Walnuts
Sprouts	Sprouted	
Spinach	Wheat	**Pasta & Noodles**
Summer Squash		Corn Pasta
Tomatoes	**Breakfast Cereals**	Quinoa Pasta
Turnips	Creamy Buckwheat	Rice Pasta
Watercress	Cream of Rye	Semolina
Winter Squash	Cream of Wheat	Soba Noodles
Zucchini	Multigrain	Udon Noodles
	Rolled Oats	Whole Wheat Pasta

Fish & Shellfish	**Oils**	**Herbs & Spices**
Bass	Coconut	Basil
Clams	Olive	Bay Leaves
Cod	Peanut	Cayenne Pepper
Flounder	Sesame	Cinnamon
Fluke	Toasted Sesame	Coriander
Haddock	Walnut	Cumin
Salmon		Oregano
Scrod	**Vinegars**	Mustard
Shrimp	Apple Cider	Rosemary
Sole	Balsamic	Sage
Tilapia	Red Wine	Sea Salt
Trout	Rice Vinegar	Shoyu
	White Wine	Tamari
Dairy		Thyme
Butter	**Spreads**	
Cheese	Almond Butter	**Canned Food**
Kefir	Fruit Jams	Beans
Milk	Peanut Butter	Sardines
Yogurt	Tahini	Salmon
		Tomato Products
Meat and Poultry	**Sweeteners**	
Beef	Fruit Juice	**Staples**
Buffalo	Granulated Cane Sugar	Bouillon Cubes
Chicken	Honey	Mayonnaise
Duck	Maple Syrup	Olives
Eggs		Stocks (boxed, canned)
Lamb	**Snacks**	
Pork	Grain Crackers	**Beverages**
Sausages	Popcorn	Almond Milk
Turkey	Tortilla Chips	Green Tea
Venison	Trail Mix	Hazelnut Milk
Wild Boar		Herbal Teas

Chapter 5

PURCHASING THE ESSENTIALS

Clients often assure me that the *real* reason they cannot get into the kitchen and cook a wholesome meal is that they do not have the proper pots and pans, or other equipment to get started. That's hogwash! The pots and pans I had (and still have) when I began cooking, nourishing, and healing my body were my mom's from the early 1970's, and were worn from many years of use. I have fond memories of a broken blue spatula that would detach from its handle every time I washed the darn thing. And, yes, I even had an old nonstick pan that is considered FORBIDDEN in most health-related practices, and for good reasons that will be explained as you read on. But, those old pots and pans and broken down spatula didn't stop me. I was on a mission to support my body, and nothing could prevent me from investing in my health. I made cooking wholesome meals a priority and ditched all the lame-duck excuses. And trust me, I had a million of them! The key to getting started is to use what you already have. The tools in your kitchen are good enough. As you continue moving forward, you can pick up any other specific things along the way as needed.

Below are some helpful purchasing suggestions for the absolute essentials that can make your time in the kitchen time well spent.

ONE GOOD KNIFE

When I first began my cooking and counseling business, I often traveled to clients' homes and taught healthful cooking techniques; or, if they had no desire to learn, I would prepare wholesome delicious meals for them. Before arriving, I would inquire if they had one good knife. The reply would always be, "Yes, of course, we have plenty of good knives." Inevitably, when I entered their kitchens and viewed the countertops filled with mounds of colorful produce that needed to be chopped, sliced, and diced, I asked the infamous question once again, "Do you have a good knife?" At that point I would be handed a large dull butter knife masquerading as a chef's knife. Attempting to slice a ripe, juicy tomato with a dull knife can quickly become a gruesome scene from a horror movie!

The one tool above all others I highly recommend purchasing is a professional chef's knife or Santoku knife (Japanese version similar to a French chef's knife, but without a pointed tip). This purchase will make your efforts in the kitchen feel like a smooth breeze instead of a harrowing hurricane! A good quality professional knife could greatly enhance your culinary experience and gustatory growth. I promise.

There is no need to buy an entire knife collection (chef's knife, paring knife, boning knife, bread knife, cleaver, and vegetable knife), and a knife block, unless of course you have the money. Then, by all means, please do. You really only need one good knife (a sharp one) to help with most of the chopping, slicing, dicing, and mincing tasks.

To purchase the perfect knife, it helps to literally try it on! I'm sure you wouldn't buy a pair of jeans straight off the rack without trying them on to see how they feel (and look) on your derriere. Think of your knife the same way and don't purchase it without trying it on.

Here's how to try on and determine which knife is best for you. At the kitchen supply store, the professional knives are usually locked up inside glass cases. I don't know if that's to protect the customer from the sharp knives, or to protect the sales staff from crazy customers that want to *try on* knives. Ask the clerk for three or four professional chef knives of varying sizes (some have longer/larger blades than others), preferably carbon steel with a full tang. The tang is the metal part of the blade that extends into the handle. Ideally, you want the metal to extend all the way through the handle. Having a "full tang" will keep your knife handle from coming loose and falling apart like my broken blue spatula.

Hold each knife, one at a time, in your hand, and feel it; lift it up, make chopping motions in the air or on the counter (be careful not to scare or cut anyone). Make sure your hand easily holds the weight of the knife. Some handles and blades are thicker and heavier than others. Find the knife that *feels* right for you. If you are comfortable holding your knife, you will be more proficient in the kitchen and less likely to cut yourself. Please do not let price dissuade you from making the best choice. This is one kitchen tool you will have for numerous years, quite possibly an entire lifetime. I've had one of my Santoku knives for over twelve years! It was a great investment, about eighty dollars at the time, and has given me many years of service. Spend anywhere from fifty to two hundred dollars, or even more, on an excellent knife. You are making an investment in your health and you are worth every penny.

TWO GOOD POTS AND PANS

For basic cooking purposes, all you really need to get started is one large frying pan and one large soup pot or six- to eight-quart stockpot, both with lids. That's it. You can accomplish almost everything with these two items. You can make soups, stocks, beans, grains, stir-fries, and blanch vegetables, sear meats, and sauté. If you have the money to buy an entire set, go for it. It surely is a worthy investment. If you don't have the funds, use the pots and pans you already have and add to your collection when you can afford it.

Traditionally, some of the best cookware has been stainless steel and cast iron, but if you don't have either, don't sweat it. Just start cooking. If you have aluminum pots and pans, it's wise to use plastic or rubber utensils on them. Scraping aluminum cookware with metal utensils can cause some of it to leach into food. Aluminum toxicity has been strongly linked with Alzheimer's disease, and other ailments.[22] Aluminum is a *reactive* metal, meaning it can react with acid or salty foods and release itself into the food product. Tomato sauce is an example of an acid food. If you are fearful of using your aluminum pots and pans, consider this: a person using aluminum-containing antacids (at about 50 mg per tablet) may consume more aluminum per day than someone using uncoated aluminum pans for cooking (ingesting approximately 3.5 mg per day).[23] If you are eating antacids on a daily basis, you don't have to worry about aluminum being leached from your pots and pans and going into your body, you're already getting plenty of it from the over-the-counter and prescription drugs.

---

[22] http://www.angelfire.com/az/sthurston/alzheimers_and_aluminum_toxicity.html
[23] http://www.dmaonline.org/fppublic/connect56.html

Cast iron is a good old-fashioned cooking choice, an ideal heat conductor, and can last a lifetime with proper care. Unfortunately, cast iron can be a pain in the buttocks as it requires special care and coating with oil to prevent rust. It's also heavy to handle (literally), so you need strong arms and wrists – this would not be an ideal choice for the elderly, physically disabled, arthritic, or weak. A nutritional benefit of using cast iron: it imparts minute traces of iron into your food. If you are anemic (low blood iron), cast iron may be a great choice. Although, if you are anemic, you may not have the strength to lift a heavy cast iron skillet.

Nonstick coatings for cookware are hard chemical plastics made with substances that can emit hazardous fumes when heated at high temperatures. These fumes have been linked with cancer, birth defects, and many other health problems. A group of scientific advisers to the Environmental Protection Agency voted unanimously to approve a recommendation that a chemical used in the manufacture of Teflon (PFOA) and other nonstick products should be considered a likely carcinogen.[24] This is serious business. If you have Teflon or other nonstick pans, do not use them to deep-fry food, and do not place them under the broiler. Never, ever use metal utensils on them (spatulas, forks, and spoons) – it increases the likelihood that you will damage the plastic coating and ingest it. Carcinogens are not appetizing and do not contribute to long-term health. When cooking with nonstick equipment, use medium or low heat, quick-cooking techniques, and plastic or wood utensils.

I prefer stainless steel for cooking. It's durable, reliable, lighter weight than cast iron, does not react negatively with foods, and is easy as

---

[24] http://www.cbsnews.com/stories/2006/02/15/tech/main1321804.shtml

heck to clean and care for. Just wash and dry – done! Stainless steel is also relatively inexpensive. I think this is an excellent choice and will give you many years of great kitchen service.

SAVVY SLOW COOKERS

For those of you working long hours away from home and still desiring fully balanced, delicious, home-cooked meals, I would highly recommend purchasing a slow cooker. Your purchase will not go to waste. There is an entire chapter dedicated to one pot meals -- The Pot of Gold -- designed specifically for people who don't have the time to cook and babysit their food, or the patience to deal with cleaning many pots and pans. It's no muss, no fuss – everything in one pot, set the timer, and go! Cooking doesn't get easier than that. Slow cookers are safe, affordable, and come in a variety of sizes. I would suggest buying a 4- or 6-quart slow cooker and spending anywhere from $29 to $100 (or more). You are worth it!

THE BIG BOARD BROUHAHA

Over the years, I've heard much controversy about which type of cutting board (plastic, rubber, wood, or glass) is best to use in the kitchen. Various studies claim that boards can retain bacteria and need to be washed with bleach or that other boards can damage knife blades. People always want to know which boards are easiest to clean. Trying to figure that stuff out is enough to drive a person right out of the kitchen and into the local pizza parlor for dinner. From a healthy chef perspective, I would advise you to purchase an old-fashioned wooden cutting board. Besides the fact that chefs have been using wooden boards for centuries, there's only one little tidbit of information I want to point out. If you have a cutting board in your kitchen, go take a look at it right now. As you can see, whether it is plastic, rubber, or wood, it probably has little nicks and scrapes on it. Those cuts come from use - chopping things on your board with a sharp knife. The question is… where do those missing pieces from the cutting board go? The answer is… they go into your food and into your body. Bottom line, wood is easier to digest than plastic, rubber, glass, or any other substance. And, if termites can survive and thrive on wood, then I can, too. Get a wooden cutting board for the sake of your health. To clean a wood board all you need to do is wipe it down with a hot sponge after each use. There is no need to use bleach or other harsh chemicals on your board – they too, will eventually be absorbed into your body. Keep raw meats separate, and don't chop raw foods (salads and vegetables) on the same board surface without cleaning it first or simply flip it over and use the opposite side. If you have the cash, you could always purchase two wooden boards of varying sizes, one for meats and one for vegetables.

OTHER HANDY UTENSILS

I love wooden spoons, rice paddles, and other wood implements. The wood feels natural in my hand and on the pots and pans. It is smooth, nonabrasive, and won't damage cooking surfaces. Wooden kitchen utensils are a great choice for use on nonstick or aluminum pots and pans.

Tongs are probably my favorite kitchen utensil. I'm only 5 feet 4 inches (on a tall day), and many of my herbs and spices are kept on the top shelf in the pantry. My tongs are an extension of my arms and help me reach those hard to get to places without having to drag out my stepladder and go mountain climbing in my kitchen. If you happen to be like me, a shorty, you might find tongs to be useful for more than just cooking. Tongs are the perfect tool for flipping meats, grabbing vegetables, tossing pastas and salads, and for pinching someone's fanny – if you happen to be cooking with someone you really like and want to grab their attention, of course.

I also have a few wire mesh strainers varying in size: a large one to rinse grains and beans and to drain pasta and vegetables; a small one for steeping bulk tea; and a round flat one to skim off foam and other impurities that rise to the top of the pot when cooking beans, grains, and meat stocks.

Slotted spoons are another handy utensil to have in the kitchen. I use slotted spoons almost daily when I'm blanching vegetables. When I want to puree or chop ingredients that are already in the soup pot, I reach for my slotted spoons. And, if I accidentally make too much sauce for my stir-fry and the veggies are drowning (hey… it happens to the best of us), a slotted spoon lets me drain the excess liquid from the vegetables before putting them onto my plate.

My next kitchen utensil, I like to sing about. We'll use the chorus to a popular Jewish holiday song called The *Dreidel*. Do you know the tune? It goes something like this… "*dreidel, dreidel, dreidel*, I made you out of clay." Just substitute the words "ladle, ladle, ladle, I like cooking all day." I love my ladle. Imagine that? I've fallen in love with a simple kitchen utensil and couldn't imagine a life without it. I mean if I had to use a regular-size spoon to get soup out of the pot, well, it would be annoying as heck and a huge waste of time! My *dreamy* ladle makes my kitchen time more efficient.

THE FABULOUS FOOD PROCESSOR

If you are cooking for large groups of people, or seriously want to reduce kitchen time, purchase a food processor. This one kitchen tool can dice, shred, julienne, puree, chop, mince – it's a real workhorse and surely a gift from the kitchen gods. There are specific discs and attachments that come with a food processor that will do the job of effortlessly chopping food for you. A food processor can cost anywhere from $90 to $900. No, that's not a typo. There are food processors that cost hundreds and even thousands of dollars, but you don't need to spend that much money. Wait for a sale at the local department store or kitchen supply shop, or go out and spend a little dough and give yourself a nice treat. The first food processor I bought cost $89 and my second $179. I have two of these timesaving tools because I teach cooking classes to a roomful of hungry folks. You may need only one to serve your kitchen needs. Always remember, the money spent in your kitchen is an investment in your health, and yep -- you guessed it -- you are worth it!

BOWL ME OVER

Sometimes I cook for two people and sometimes I cook for twenty or more. That means I use a lot of different size bowls in the kitchen. Having various mixing bowls available allows me to combine ingredients neatly and easily. I know it may sound like a "no-brainer" but, if you mix something (salad, pasta, or dressing) in a small bowl, you could spill ingredients all over the counter, make a mess, and create more work for yourself. You'll have to spend extra time on clean-up duty, and would probably get angry at me for forcing you into that darn dirty kitchen in the first place. I can see it now... your clenched fist raised high in the air, while you're cleaning up a nasty oil spill, "Damn that Andrea Beaman and her blasted cookbook!" The simple and easy way for you to keep your kitchen clean, and continue to have positive feelings about this healthy chef, is to purchase a set of glass or stainless steel mixing bowls of various sizes that neatly stack into each other and won't take up much space in your cabinets. The right size mixing bowl will help keep your ingredients contained. Less mess equals less kitchen time. Life is good and we're the best of friends once again.

STORE YOUR STUFF

Last but not least, you are going to need storage containers. In upcoming chapters, I'm going to teach you how to cook in bulk to help save both time and money. Having delicious homemade food available is a great way to get healthy, and you are going to need somewhere to store this savory stuff. The better your storage containers, the longer food can keep fresh. If you put food into the refrigerator and cover it with foil or plastic wrap, air can seep in. It is the oxidation process that ages food and makes it go bad. Metal, glass, or plastic containers with airtight tops make great storage units. I even use glass jars with screw-tops to store some of my yummy vittles. After I use up a store-bought item that has been packaged in a glass jar, I simply soak the jar overnight in hot water to peel off the label. By the morning, I have a new food storage container without having to pay for it. Nice! You can use the extra money you saved to shop for more delicious food. Or… you could save some extra cash each week, and then go out and buy a fun and flirty outfit to fit your fabulous new and improved physique. Ooh la la.

Now that we've got the *bare essentials* of your kitchen and pantry squared away, we can start doing a little cooking. Yeah, baby! Are you ready for this culinary adventure? It's not as big an expenditure as it may seem. I know between the shopping for ingredients and kitchen utensils, you may be thinking you're going to be broke. It's not true. I'll show you how to save big bucks in the following chapter.

Chapter 6

SAVE BIG BUCKS!

One of the best ways to save big bucks is by cooking healthful and delicious meals at home. I bet you think I'm just saying that because I love to cook and want to encourage you to do the same. Nope. I'm saying it because it's true! Purchasing and cooking food at home can save you some serious cabbage (money). Check out these financial facts:

BULK IT UP, BABY!

Many health food stores carry "bulk" food items. These include a wide variety of whole grains and grain products, beans, nuts, seeds, dried fruits, snacks, and other foods that are not packaged but are kept in large bulk bins. Bulk foods generally cost less than packaged foods because you are not paying for the "designer" bags and containers they are kept in. The container inevitably winds up in the garbage at some point anyway, so why dish out the extra dough? It's not as if someone will peer into your pantry, notice the bulk-bought raisins stored in a glass jar, and say, "Hey, those raisins are *not* in a pretty package!" And, the next thing you know you have been mysteriously blacklisted from the local community or PTA meetings. Oh the ridicule!

C'mon… who the heck cares what anyone thinks? Don't let pride get in the way of making smart purchasing choices. The bottom line: bulk items cost less and can help save money. All you need to do is store bulk-bought items in either plastic or glass containers to keep them fresh and safe from hungry closet critters.

And, if you want to save *more money,* you don't even have to purchase storage containers for these bulk items. As I mentioned in a previous chapter, you can reuse any jar or bottle in your refrigerator or pantry. After finishing a jar of pickles, sauerkraut, pasta sauce, or other bottled item, instead of throwing out the container, recycle it for your own use. Soak the jar overnight in warm water to remove the label. Once it is cleaned, you have a handy-dandy container at no extra cost. I have many recycled bottles in varying sizes. I even recycle jelly jars to store delicious dressings and sauces.

Let's take a look at some of the savings you could make by purchasing bulk food items:

PRODUCT	**BULK COST**	**PACKAGED COST**	**SAVINGS**
Dried Beans	$2.29 per lb.	$3.62 per lb.	**$1.33 per lb.**
Rolled Oats	$1.40 per lb.	$2.76 per lb.	**$1.36 per lb.**
Cranberries	$10.99 per lb.	$17.16 per lb.	**$6.17 per lb.**
Walnuts	$12.99 per lb.	$20.77 per lb.	**$7.78 per lb.**

Prices may vary from store to store, but the savings are still quite significant. Buying in bulk is an easy way to save money.

A CSA CAN SAVE THE DAY

There are many great reasons to buy into a Community Supported Agriculture (CSA); but for the purposes of this book, it's just about one of the *smartest* investments you can make. For example, I belong to a CSA in Manhattan where I purchase a share in an organic farm at the beginning of each year. Every week, the farmer drops off my share of the harvest at a designated pick-up site. "I pay $495 (not including meat and eggs) for approximately twenty-four weeks of produce. That comes out to $20 per week for two bags of food that could include two onions, one bunch of carrots, broccoli, Swiss chard, a head of cabbage, five sweet red peppers, four frying peppers, three eggplants, two jalapeno peppers, butternut winter squash, one bunch of beets, fresh basil, eight to ten small potatoes, and two leeks (this is a sample week, the harvest varies weekly). That's a large quantity of organic food for a small price. I could pay that same $20 (or more) for one meal and a cup of tea at a local restaurant.[25] Buying from a local CSA saves me a bundle of cash and aligns my body with the seasons and the environment, keeping me healthy at the same time. The produce from the farm in upstate New York is local, which means it was picked at the peak of maturity (containing the most nutrients), has spent less time in transit, and supports my community and the entire country! The future of our food system depends on supporting local farmers so we can feed ourselves as a nation and not rely on imports for our needs. Eating locally is imperative for our health and the health of the entire planet and is a point I really want to drive home… so I just may mention it in every darn chapter. Locating a participating CSA near you is easy. Go to localharvest.org, justfood.org, or eatwellguide.org, and punch in your zip code. A list of participating CSAs available in your area will pop up. Choose one, sign up, and send a check to your local farmer. It's that easy to get started eating well and saving BIG bucks. Life is delicious!

CASH IN WITH REAL VITAMINS AND MINERALS

Before taking charge of my health and diet, I spent thousands of dollars buying vitamin and mineral supplements to help make up for my

---

[25] The Whole Truth Eating and Recipe Guide, By Andrea Beaman, 2006 p.65

dietary deficiencies and lack of good nutrition. The supplement industry is raking in millions (probably more like billions) of dollars annually, preying on folks like you and me who are concerned about health. I used to believe supplementation could help heal my ailments and make up for my lack of proper nourishment. Boy… was I mistaken. I wasted a lot of money chasing wild claims and may have harmed my body in the process, too. I know I've mentioned information about supplements in a previous chapter, but it's a point I want to get across. According to the Journal of the American Medical Association, antioxidant vitamins increased a person's risk of dying by up to 16 percent. The University of Washington found that vitamin E elevates lung cancer risk, and researchers at the National Cancer Institute found that men who took more than one multivitamin daily had higher rates of prostate cancer.[26] According to the Canadian Medical Association Journal, below is a list of popular supplements and their toxic effects:[27]

SUPPLEMENT	POTENTIAL TOXIC EFFECTS
Vitamin A	Hepatoxicity (liver damage), increased risk of hip fracture
Beta carotene	Increased risk of lung cancer, yellowing of skin, diarrhea, arthralgias (arthritis)
Vitamin C	Diarrhea, gastric upset
Vitamin D	Calcification of the soft tissue
Vitamin E	Nausea, vomiting, diarrhea, headache, fatigue, blurred vision
Vitamin B6	Sensory neuropathy, ataxia (lack of coordination and muscle movements)
Vitamin B3	Vasodilation, gastrointestinal upset, hyperglycemia

[26] http://www.rd.com/living-healthy/are-vitamins-really-that-good-for-you-/article46647.html

[27] http://www.cmaj.ca/cgi/content/full/169/1/47/T127

These are just a select few of the more common supplements and their toxic effects. *All* supplements, when taken in excess, can have negative effects on the body.

One important thing to remember is that animals in the wild do not need supplements to thrive -- and neither do humans. We are a part of nature, and the wholesome food naturally provided by our environment contains all the elements we need in perfect balance (fiber, water, protein, vitamins, minerals, and carbohydrates). Our body uses what it needs and discards the waste. Overdoses of isolated supplements accumulate and wreak havoc on our system. In the short term, supplements may do some good; but in the long term, they can cause serious harm.

There are better and more delicious ways to get the vitamins and minerals your body needs without the toxic side effects. On the following page is a chart of some of the many vitamins and minerals and their natural food sources. And, in upcoming chapters, I will show you how to make those foods taste totally scrumptious.

VITAMIN AND MINERAL FOODS[28]

VITAMIN/MINERAL	FOOD SOURCES
Vitamin A	Carrots, sweet potatoes, broccoli, dark leafy greens
Vitamin D	Salmon, fatty fish, eggs, sunshine
Vitamin B12	Shellfish, meat, fish, poultry, eggs
Chromium	Poultry, meat, whole grains
Copper	Beets, molasses, beans, nuts
Iron	Organ meats, eggs, meat, poultry
Magnesium	Whole grains, beans
Manganese	Nuts, seeds, whole grains, seaweed
Selenium	Whole grains, meat
Iodine	Seafood, sea vegetables, sea salt
Vitamin C	Berries, fruit, green vegetables
Vitamin E	Vegetable oils, nuts, seeds, eggs, organ meats, whole grains
Vitamin K	Dark leafy green vegetables, whole grains, asparagus (most vitamin K is synthesized in the intestines by our friendly bacteria)
Folic Acid (folate)	Asparagus, green leafy vegetables, whole grains, meat
Calcium	Dairy food, salmon and sardines with bones, green vegetables, almonds, sesame seeds, tofu
Phosphorus	Found in most foods (deficiency of this vitamin is rare)
Potassium	Fish, legumes, meat, poultry, vegetables, apricots, sea vegetables, nuts, raisins, spinach
Silicon	Alfalfa, beets, green veggies, whole grains
Sulfur	Garlic, cruciferous vegetables, eggs, onions
Zinc	Meat, eggs, beans, whole grains

Stop wasting money on costly supplements and purchase wholesome, natural foods instead. Your body will love you for it!

---

[28] Prescription For Nutritional Healing, Phyllis A. Balch, CNC, Penguin Books

PRESCRIPTION FOR LIVING

While we're on the subject of wasting money, let's talk about prescription drugs. I wrote about this important subject in my first book, *The Whole Truth, How I Naturally Reclaimed My Health and You can Too*, and will reiterate it here. Pharmaceutical drugs do *not* cure ailments. The drugs that big pharma are peddling to us merely cover up symptoms without getting to the root cause of the problem. If we do not get to the cause of the ailment, there will always be an underlying imbalance or dysfunction progressively growing worse the longer it is covered up.

Pharmaceuticals drugs are expensive, and buying into this drug scam is one of the biggest money wasters, contributing to more problems without real solutions. We are being flimflammed and scammed out of our hard earned bucks, and essentially out of our health.

Some doctors (the "drug dealers") will attempt to make you feel small and convince you that your body is not capable of healing itself. This is total bullcrap! The human body is an amazing creation and capable of many things – including healing itself. Take your power back and JUST SAY NO TO DRUGS! I highly encourage you to stand up for yourself and take action. Grab those prescription medications, dig a hole in your backyard, and bury them deep in the dirt where they can't harm anyone, and say a prayer for the earthworms. I would also suggest that when you get to the doctor's office tell your physician to stick that prescription note pad where the sun doesn't shine. I'm just sayin'…

Okay… now, I'm stepping off my soapbox (momentarily, of course) and getting back to food, glorious food, to show you how to save your health, and save more money, too!

THE WHOLE KIT AND KABOODLE

One of my favorite things to do (besides hug and kiss my nephews!), is dine out with friends, family, and loved ones, and be served a fantastic four-star meal. But, I do not do that daily because it can get quite expensive.

For example, the cost of one chicken entrée at an average restaurant can range from $15 to $25. For that money, I would receive one meal, possibly two if I were to take home leftovers. But, how often do leftovers really make it home from the restaurant? Not often.

On the other hand, if I purchased one entire chicken (naturally raised), it would cost approximately $9 to $20. This would provide two breasts, two legs, two thighs, two wings, the liver, heart, and neck (although, I recently bought a few chickens that were missing these valuable internal organs and I felt totally ripped off!), and leftover carcass and meat to make a rich stock. Essentially, for less than the cost of one entrée at a restaurant, I could create eight to ten meals, or more, from one chicken. Let's do the math: ten restaurant entrees could cost anywhere from $150 to $250 compared to a $15 whole chicken purchase. Holy cow! Or more appropriately, Holy Chicken! The savings could be HUGE.

Saving mounds of money is a cinch when you purchase a whole animal as often as possible. These savings work the same way when you buy a whole turkey, duck, goose, fish, or larger animal like a pig or cow (if you have room for the animal in your freezer). I actually know only *one* person who has room for an entire cow in his freezer. Let's stick with smaller animals for the at-home chef. In the chapters that follow, we are going to begin cooking and I will teach you how to make the most of your whole purchases, beginning with hearty stocks that contain an abundance of vitamins and minerals that are good nutrition for your bones and the rest of your beautiful body.

BROWN BAG IT

Packing homemade food for lunch can save big bucks, too. For example, at a popular bakery/restaurant chain, a Chicken Curry Salad Sandwich costs $9 (not including tax and tip). On the other hand, an entire loaf of whole grain bread can be purchased for less than $4. We can use the meat from a store-bought whole chicken (as described in the previous paragraph) and create eight sandwiches or more. The massive amounts of money saved over one week, or one month, or one year, could surely add up to an early retirement plan.

Trust me… cooking meals at home can save us TONS of money. Home cooking has more benefits than just saving some dough though; it nourishes us physically and emotionally and brings the family together for meals again. So c'mon, save some money and save your health. Now… it's time to get that apron on and start cooking!

Chapter 7

FROM PORRIDGE TO PROSPERITY

No ifs, ands, or buts about it: breakfast is *the* most important meal of the day. If your goal is to invest wisely in your body, it's imperative that you make time for a nourishing breakfast. I realize I may sound like a nagging wife or mom; I don't care. Moms and wives (and dads and other caretakers) instinctively know loved ones need proper nourishment to start the day. If you are the modern American who typically skedaddles out of the house without eating breakfast, it's time to sit your butt down and listen up!

"Breakfast" literally means to break the fast. When we sleep at night, we are fasting (not eating food) and not consciously moving our muscles; this causes a lowering of our body temperature.[29] In the morning it's best to break-fast with something warm to help heat the body and slowly bring it up to speed (metabolic speed). Eating something ice cold (think frozen smoothie or cold cereal with milk) requires extra effort from the body to stoke our digestive fire. Over time, consistently eating iced or cold food in the morning can exhaust energy reserves. Eating cold food for breakfast is what we Americans do most often.

Many cultures around the world traditionally ate *warm* soft porridges or gruel, and a variety of soups or congees made from cooked rice, corn, rye, and other grains combined with water, animal milk, or coconut milk for breakfast. Some heartier breakfast options included

---

[29] http://www.anti-aging-guide.com/34bodytemp.php

eggs, bacon, and sausages. And, on a lighter note, warm tea or coffee with whole grain bread and butter was another simple way to start the day. Below is a quick overview of some *traditional* breakfasts from around the globe:

Africa – fermented porridge called Ogi, made from corn and milk.
Britain and Ireland – grain porridge, eggs, bacon, black pudding (sausage prepared with boiled animal blood – *this is also a favorite breakfast treat for vampires*).
Burma – fried rice with boiled peas, buttered naan (flat bread), or fried chapattis (unleavened whole grain wheat or millet bread).
China – congee (rice boiled in 10 to 12 times the amount of water), salted eggs, steamed buns with meat or vegetables, soup, and warm tea.
Denmark – soft boiled eggs, warm bread with butter or cheese.
Greece – coffee, spanakopita (spinach and cheese pastry), bougatsa (cheese, minced meat, and phyllo dough).
India – steamed rice with coconut milk (Ganji), fermented rice with dal (made from lentils or other legumes), warm breads with fresh butter and tea.
Japan - okayu (rice boiled in 5 times the amount of water), eggs, pickles, miso, seafood, warm tea.
Pakistan – nihari (stew made from beef or lamb) eaten with naan bread and butter.
Philippines – garlic fried rice or scrambled eggs.
Russia – kasha, eggs, meats, whole grain breads with butter, oatmeal.
Scandinavia – whole grain porridges, eggs, cured meat, whole grain bread.
Scotland – whole grain porridge, oats, boiled eggs.
South America – tortillas (flat bread made from maize or wheat), arepas (bread made from corn), meat, beans, coffee, bread with butter.
Thai – jok, a boiled rice dish with fish, pickles, or dried shredded pork.
United States – corn grits, oatmeal, grain porridge, eggs, bacon, ham, fried potatoes, warm biscuits, or whole grain bread with butter.

It seems all over the world, *warm* breakfast was an important start to the day. Even in fairy tales, Goldilocks and the Three Bears had a piping bowl of hot porridge on the morning menu. These types of breakfast foods ready our digestive system for absorption and assimilation of nutrients.

In the past one hundred years or so, we have radically altered that traditional warm morning start and now begin the day with the exact opposite: frozen smoothies, hard cereals with ice-cold milk; or worse yet… skip breakfast entirely. Egads! This can be a recipe for disaster.

The types of breakfast we choose can either support us in starting the day or make us want to crawl right back into bed. And, for those folks suffering with digestive disorders (Crohn's, colitis, IBS, etc.), a cold breakfast cereal may make them want to crawl right into the nearest hospital! How on earth could an innocent little breakfast flake do so much damage?

Cereal flakes were originally created by Will Keith Kellogg. "In 1894, Kellogg was trying to improve the diet of hospital patients. He was searching for a digestible bread substitute using the process of boiling wheat. Kellogg accidentally left a pot of boiled wheat to stand and the wheat became tempered (softened). When Kellogg rolled the tempered or softened wheat and let it dry, each grain of wheat emerged as a large thin flake. The flakes turned out to be a tasty cereal."[30] Had cereal flakes remained the way Kellogg originally created, they may still be a nutritious option. But, the way they are processed today is downright disease-promoting. "Boxed breakfast cereals are made by an extrusion process, in which little flakes and shapes are formed at extreme high temperatures and pressures. Extrusion processing destroys many valuable nutrients in grains, causes fragile oil to become rancid and renders certain proteins

[30] http://inventors.about.com/library/inventors/blcereal.htm

toxic."[31] Beginning the day with rancid oil and toxic protein is not advisable or appetizing.

For the sake of convenience and time, cold boxed cereals took the place of warm homemade whole grain porridges. This unhealthful takeover may have occurred when women stopped cooking in the kitchen and started working outside the home. Without mom cooking breakfast, the kiddies and the men were left to fend for themselves. Our loved ones need nutritional guidance, and they're certainly not going to get it reading the back of a highly processed cereal box.

Recently, a client came for nutritional guidance. During his session I recommended a program that included many types of foods including "whole grains."

When I mentioned whole grains, he became enthusiastic, sat straight up in his chair, and stated, "That's great! I already eat whole grains every morning."

"Really? What do you eat?"

He smiled and said, "Cheerios!"

"Well," I said, "that's great… and you've got the right idea, but… maybe not the right product. Cheerios aren't *really* a whole grain."

"Oh yes, they are" he defended. "It says so right on the box."

And, he was right. It said so right on the box. The makers of many breakfast cereals have begun adding the words "Whole Grain" onto the packaging to make them seem like a better food choice. But, they are not really. On a recent visit to the supermarket, I discovered Lucky Charms, Cocoa Puffs, and Cookie Crisp (and many other highly processed cereals) stamped with a **"Whole Grain Guaranteed"** label. Besides

---

[31] Nourishing Traditions, By Sally Fallon, New Trends Publishing 2001, p. 454

being a very distant-cousin-once-removed from the whole grain family, the ingredients that make Lucky Charms "magically delicious" are various types of sugar, corn syrup, and dextrose (more sugar). And, as far as Cocoa Puffs and Cookie Crisp go… well… let's just say I believe they are the equivalent to "Crack in a Box." The glycemic index on these and other highly refined sugar-coated breakfast cereals is so high it can have kids (and adults) bouncing off the walls, unable to concentrate at school or work, and doped up on Attention Deficit Disorder drugs.

Many of these cold hard breakfast cereals can inhibit the process of digestion and eventually lead to debilitating digestive disorders. According to traditional Chinese medicine, excessive consumption of cold food, raw food, and iced drinks weakens the spleen and contracts the intestines, causing blood stagnation. Blood is fuel (food) for our entire system. Blood stagnation can create a breeding ground for many diseases. Eating cold cereal for breakfast, a cold salad for lunch, and a frozen yogurt for dessert, as many people do, could lead to serious health problems.

This does not mean *never* eat cold hard cereal with milk or a morning smoothie ever again. Just try not to eat it on a daily basis. I have discovered that when clients transition from eating cold breakfast foods to something warm and nourishing, they generally feel more energized, less bloated, and tend to lose weight easily.

For those of you doing a mad dash out of the house in the morning without eating breakfast - yikes! It's time to slow down and enjoy a warm bowl of morning porridge; or, at the very least, sit down to a cup of tea with whole grain bread and a little pat of butter. Skipping breakfast contributes to increased levels of the stress hormone cortisol and to mood swings, and has been linked to higher rates of obesity. And, get this --

skipping breakfast has also been associated with many other bad habits: lack of exercise, smoking, and caffeine/drug/alcohol addiction.[32] Holy Whole Grain Porridge, Goldilocks -- imagine that! Running out of the house without taking the time to properly nourish the body is a bad habit that should be kicked ASAP.

The American Dietetic Association's Complete Food and Nutrition Guide states that breakfast is imperative because "the brain needs a fresh supply of glucose, its main energy source, because it has no stored reserves." Studies have shown that people who eat breakfast perform better at both work and school, have a better attitude, higher productivity, more strength and endurance, and improved concentration and memory.[33] Wow! This means we have the opportunity to begin the day smarter, stronger, healthier, more focused, and even more fabulous. What could be better than that?

Rise and shine – it's time for breakfast!

---

[32] http://www.medicalnewstoday.com/articles/4004.php

[33] http://books.google.com/books?id=1PTsJgQI7w0C&pg=PA235&lpg=PA235&dq=skipping+breakfast+stress+hormone&source=web&ots=Bvt6k0oug9&sig=bN33F-tKX0uiuyzAERjtzAeExIE&hl=en&sa=X&oi=book_result&resnum=7&ct=result#PPA235,M1

BREAKFAST PORRIDGE

Porridge refers to hot cereal grains prepared with water or milk and cooked until thick, creamy, and delicious. Softening the grains renders them more digestible. Any grain can be used to make porridge: corn, wheat, rye, oats, millet, rice, barley, spelt, kamut, buckwheat, and farro. You can use the recipe below with *any* leftover grain. For this porridge, I use leftover rice. If you're not in the habit of cooking large enough portions of food to have leftover grain available, don't sweat it. On your next shopping excursion to the health food store or market, purchase cracked grain or whole grain breakfast cereals. Read the ingredient list to make sure they are *really* whole grain and not puffed flaked cereals. It may say whole grain or cracked grain plus salt and nothing else. Some store-bought examples include Cream of Buckwheat, Cream of Rye, Multigrain Porridge, Cream of Wheat, and Cream of Rice. Follow the instructions on the box and you can have a piping hot bowl of porridge in 5 to 10 minutes, depending on the grain.

1 cup cooked brown rice
2 cups water (or milk)
2 tablespoons dried raisins
Dash cinnamon
½ cup walnuts, dry-roasted (see following page)
2 to 3 tablespoons yogurt

Procedure:

1. In a medium pot, bring rice, water, raisins, and cinnamon to a boil. Reduce heat to medium.
2. Cover and cook for 7 to 10 minutes, or until creamy.
3. Remove from heat, and serve topped with walnuts and yogurt.

ROASTING NUTS

To roast walnuts, or any other nut:

1. Preheat oven to 350° F.
2. Place raw nuts onto a baking sheet.
3. Roast in the oven, shaking the pan occasionally, for 8 to 10 minutes, or until lightly browned.

TOASTING NUTS

To toast nuts on top of the stove:

1. Heat a skillet over low heat.
2. Place raw nuts into the skillet without any oil.
3. Gently shake or move the nuts frequently to prevent them from burning.
4. The nuts will become lightly browned and release a "nutty fragrance" when they are done (approximately 10 to 12 minutes).

CONGEE

In many countries, there is some variation of congee (jook, jok, ganji, okayu) or Chinese rice gruel (aka **hsi-fan**) traditionally eaten for breakfast. If you have the time, try this simple version of congee which is prepared from scratch, beginning with the whole grain (not leftover cooked grain as used in the previous recipe). Some folks use rice plus water, coconut milk, or animal milk: goat, sheep, cow, or llama!

1 cup whole grain brown rice
5 to 6 cups water or milk
1 teaspoon sea salt

Procedure:

1. In a medium pot, bring rice and water to a boil.
2. Add salt, cover, and reduce heat to simmer.
3. Cook 2 to 3 hours.

Additions: During the last ½ hour of cooking, you can add more ingredients such as:

Tofu

Meat

Fish

Vegetables

Seaweed

Nuts

Fruits

Or anything you think would be enjoyable in your version of congee.

MISO SALMON SOUP

Soup for breakfast? Yes, this is a magnificent way to begin the day. Soup is warm and gentle on the digestive system. I especially love soups in the wintertime, but can certainly wake up and slurp them down all year round.

½ onion, peeled and cut into thin crescents
2 to 3 cups water or fish stock
3 to 4 ounces salmon or other fish (can use drained canned salmon)
2 kale leaves, cut into bite-size pieces
1 tablespoon sweet miso per cup of water
2 to 3 scallions, minced

Procedure:

1. In a medium pot, bring onion and water to a boil.
2. Reduce heat to medium.
3. Add fish and kale, and cook, covered, for 2 to 3 minutes.
4. Dilute miso in a small amount of water (can use cooking water from the pot) and add to the soup.
5. Continue cooking on low heat for 2 to 3 minutes.
6. Pour into individual bowls and garnish with scallions.

OATS & ALMONDS

There are many delicious oat options: whole oat groats, cracked oats, and rolled oats. Oat groats take approximately three hours to cook, so they may not be ideal for a busy person. Rolled oats are quicker at seven to ten minutes, and cracked oats cook in about twenty to thirty minutes. My dad taught me this quick-cooking version of cracked oats, which are also known as steel cut oats. Before bedtime, bring the oats and water up to a boil, then turn off the heat, and let them sit overnight. The oats soak in the warm water and cook through the night while you're sleeping. In the morning, all you need to do is turn up the heat for 2 to 3 minutes. Nice! It seems that not only is dad handsome, generous, witty, and extremely likable, he's a genius too!

1¾ cups water
½ cup cracked oats
Pinch sea salt
¼ cup dried cranberries
Dash cinnamon
¼ cup slivered almonds, roasted
¼ cup almond milk

Procedure:

1. In a medium pot, bring water and oats to a boil.
2. Cover pot and turn off the heat.
3. Let oats and hot water sit, covered, overnight.
4. In the morning, add salt, cranberries, and cinnamon.
5. Turn on heat to high, and bring back up to a boil.
6. Cover and cook on medium heat 2 to 3 minutes.
7. Serve topped with almonds and almond milk.

SAVORY OATS & SAUSAGE

Many people begin their day with "sweet" oats or other sweetened cereal grain. This recipe is for all the "savory" type people.

1½ cups water
½ cup rolled oats
1 tablespoon butter
Pinch sea salt
Pinch cinnamon
1 teaspoon olive oil or other fat

1 pork, chicken, or turkey sausage link, diced
1 tablespoon sauerkraut or other type of pickled food
Parsley, minced

Procedure:

1. In a medium pot, bring water, oats, butter, salt and cinnamon, to a boil.
2. Reduce heat to low, cover, and cook 6 to 8 minutes.
3. While oats are cooking, in a separate skillet, heat olive oil and add diced sausage
4. Cook sausage according to directions on package.
5. Place oats in individual bowls and top with sausage and sauerkraut.
6. Garnish with parsley.

RAVISHING ROLLED OATS

I love oats in the morning. Maybe it's my Scottish, English, and Irish heritage, or maybe it's just because they are satisfying and delicious. Many clients have told me they "can't stand oatmeal - ew!" They cite it as boring and bland. Of course it is… if it's consumed without any flavorful accoutrements. I advise clients to dress up their oats. It's similar to the way we magically transform a boring black dress into a fabulous outfit: add a sparkling bracelet, a flirty necklace, a shiny brooch, and a gorgeous pair of high-heeled red pumps. Zowee! What a difference accessories can make. If you want your oats to be fabulous, dress them up with flavorful accessories.

1½ cups water
1/3 cup rolled oats
Pinch sea salt
½ apple or pear, cored and diced (in the winter, mostly)
OR ¼ cup fresh blueberries or blackberries (in the summer, mostly)
¼ cup yogurt, almond milk, or other milk
1 tablespoon maple syrup
1/3 cup walnuts, or other nuts, toasted
¼ cup sunflower seeds, toasted

Procedure:

1. In a medium pot, bring water and oats to a boil. Stir in salt.
2. During the cold months, add an apple or pear and cook with the oats on medium heat for 7 to 10 minutes.

In the warmer months, cook the oats 7 to 10 minutes, and then *top* with fresh berries at the end of cooking.

3. Mix together the yogurt and maple syrup and put a dollop or two on top of the oatmeal. Garnish with crunchy toasted walnuts and seeds.

Not only does that bland boring oatmeal now look more appetizing, it also contains additional healthful properties from the nuts and fruit. And, it has exciting textures (creamy and crunchy), heightened flavor, and sultry sweetness. Ooh la la!

POACHED EGGS

The poor innocent little egg was beaten up so badly in the early 1980s during the no-fat, low-fat, eliminate-cholesterol craze. At the time, researchers warned us that cholesterol and fat in the egg yolk were bad for our health. Current research proves the once-dreaded yolk is actually the most healthful part of the egg! Yolks contain lutein and zeaxanthin (both powerful healing carotenoids), lecithin (an essential fatty acid), and vitamins A, D, E, and K. I had a client who would consume three egg whites for breakfast and couldn't understand why she had *intense* fat cravings in the afternoon. She confessed to sometimes eating a third of a jar of peanut butter in one sitting! Egads! I suggested she eat one or two entire eggs (with the yolk) instead of just egg whites. Within a few days, her fat cravings had diminished, and by the end of the week, had disappeared entirely. Moral of the story: eat the whole egg! If you don't, the body will naturally search for the fat elsewhere. The recipe below is my favorite way to eat eggs. It's quick and simple.

Whole grain bread (one slice per egg)
2 to 3 cups water
1 teaspoon white distilled, apple cider, brown rice, or other light colored vinegar
1 or two eggs per person
Butter
Sea salt
Freshly ground black pepper

Procedure:

1. Put bread in the toaster or oven.
2. In a small pot, bring water to a boil.
3. Add vinegar.
4. Reduce heat to medium-low.
5. Crack egg into a small bowl.
6. Gently drop the egg from the bowl into the water.
7. Cook three minutes for a soft egg and four or five minutes for a firm egg.
8. Butter the toast and place it on a plate.
9. Use a slotted spoon or other utensil to gently lift the egg from the water.
10. Place egg on top of buttered toast and sprinkle with salt and pepper to taste.

Eggs are an excellent source of concentrated fat and protein and can be fully satisfying. If eaten in *excess*, sometimes eggs (as with any food) can congest our systems, contributing to liver or gallbladder stagnation. I always suggest clients begin with *one* egg and gauge if they are still hungry afterwards. If they are, it's easy to prepare a second or third egg in three to five minutes or less.

SCRAMBLED EGGS CON VEGGIES

When my nephews come to visit, we make scrambled eggs in the morning. I usually add diced vegetables and fresh herbs to the eggs, and believe it or not… one or two of those "dreaded" veggies accidentally make it into their little digestive systems. That makes this aunt very happy!

1 tablespoon olive oil or other fat (chicken fat, butter)
¼ cup blanched broccoli florets (to blanch, simply drop into boiling water for 1 to 2 minutes and drain)
2 scallions, minced
1 tablespoon butter
1 or 2 eggs per person, beaten
Sea salt
¼ cup grated raw milk cheddar cheese
Freshly ground black pepper

Procedure:

1. Heat oil in a frying pan and sauté broccoli and scallions in the oil for 1 to 2 minutes.
2. Add butter to the same pan with the vegetables.
3. Add eggs and a few pinches of sea salt.
4. Reduce heat to medium-low.
5. As the texture of the eggs firms up, use a wooden spoon or spatula to pull the eggs away from the sides of the pan.
6. Continue pulling the eggs from the sides of the pan to the center until the eggs are firm but still moist.
7. Serve topped with grated cheese and pepper.

Use any vegetables you enjoy to help boost the beneficial properties of the eggs. Or, use no veggies at all. Eggs are just as healthful exactly the way they are without the veggies… just don't tell my nephews.

Variations of Scrambled Eggs with Vegetables:

- Sauté chopped red bell pepper and chopped onion instead of using blanched broccoli florets
- Sauté chopped shallots, diced ham, and shredded Swiss cheese
- Sauté chopped leeks and sliced mushrooms
- Garnish with minced chives or other fresh herbs

CREAMY POLENTA AND FRIED EGGS

This breakfast option may take a little longer than the average breakfast (about 30 minutes), but it's worth it!

1¾ cups water
½ cup polenta
Sea salt
2 tablespoons butter
Olive oil
2 eggs (1 per serving)
Freshly ground black pepper

Procedure:

1. In a medium pot, bring water to a boil.
2. Add polenta, ¼ teaspoon salt, and butter.
3. Lower heat to simmer. Cook, stirring occasionally, for 25 minutes, or until polenta is thick and creamy.
4. In a skillet, heat olive oil over medium heat.
5. Crack eggs into a bowl and gently add them to the skillet, keeping yolks intact.
6. Sprinkle a pinch of salt and pepper on top of each egg.
7. Cook eggs until lightly browned and crispy around the edges.
8. Place polenta into individual bowls and top with a fried egg.

Chapter 8

INVESTING IN GOOD STOCK

Have you ever heard the expression "he or she comes from good stock"? It means the individual came from a family with excellent physical constitutions that included vibrant health, strong bones, and good teeth. Your constitution is the strength you are born with and has been passed down to you from your ancestors. If your constitution is strong, you can thank your parents, grandparents, great grandparents, and all of your ancestors for their wise lifestyle and diet choices. On the other hand, if your constitution is poor and you are prone to chronic sickness and are easily fatigued, you have permission to slap your relatives at the next family reunion!

A strong constitution is one of the many reasons Grandma Moses or Uncle George (George Burns, that is) could drink and smoke excessively, and party 'til the cows came home, and still live to the ripe old age of 101 with little or no consequences. Those folks are living off the strength of their ancestral lineage.

Unfortunately, many more young people are developing chronic and debilitating sicknesses earlier in life. This means, with each passing generation, we are growing weaker. Our "good stock" is plummeting while illness and disease are on the rise. To offset this current imbalance, we need to invest in good stock, literally.

Stock is the liquid gold created through the alchemy of cooking animal bones. Our ancestors did not waste natural resources as food was scarce at times. They used every part of the animal, not just the prime cuts. Bones, feet, skin, and scraps too were boiled in water, creating a vitamin- and mineral-rich liquid. Interestingly, folklore in many cultures alluded to bone stock as an all-around panacea for anyone sick or weak. It was traditionally used to cure flu, colds, digestive problems, bone loss, joint pain, skin disorders, muscles weakness, blood deficiency, and many other ailments.[34]

My father grew up in America during the great depression in the 1900s. He told me a story of how his mother used to feed the entire family (five children and two parents) on very little money. She would go to the butcher shop and purchase bones--just bones, no meat, for mere pennies. Then she purchased a single head of cabbage and a couple of potatoes. With those three ingredients, plus water, she made soup. That simple bone and vegetable soup not only nourished the family so they could survive the depression, but also kept them quite healthy and strong.

Stock contains a wealth of nutrients including gelatin, marrow, cartilage, collagen, amino acids, minerals, and trace minerals. Besides being nutritionally beneficial, stock imparts a rich hearty flavor that lingers seductively on the tongue and is, therefore, used in many professional kitchens as the base for soups, sauces, and gravies.

One of the most amazing attributes of this uber-nourishing liquid is that it is practically effortless to prepare. No joke. Once you acquire the bones, the preparation consists of combining them with water, vegetables, and seasonings, then simmering them for many hours without having to babysit the darn pot. If the idea of leaving stock cooking for hours on the stove makes you nervous, it would be wise to purchase a slow cooker. A

[34] http://findarticles.com/p/articles/mi_m0ISW/is_259-260/ai_n10299306/pg_1

slow cooker cooks your food, unattended, for ten to twelve hours and shuts off automatically when finished. We'll elaborate on slow cookers in the *Pot of Gold* chapter. The most labor-intensive part of the stock-making process is procuring the bones or other parts (like feet) at the onset, and preparing it for storage at the end. Stock must be strained, cooled, skimmed, and put into freezer-safe containers.

Trust me -- making a savory bone stock one or two times per month is well worth your time and effort. You and your family will feel the benefits all the way down to your bones. Many folks spend hundreds (even thousands) of dollars on glucosamine and chondroitin supplements to help heal their arthritic and bone woes. Stock contains these elements, organically.

Increasing your family's good stock begins with purchasing an entire animal (chicken, duck, turkey, pheasant, fish, cow, goat, lamb, pig, wild boar, or deer). My friends, Jeannie and Anthony DelGreco, and a couple other families bought an entire cow and then had it butchered and split up among them. That's a smart way to purchase food. It reduced their meat bill considerably and fed quite a few families. If you have the room or an extra freezer, to save some money, think about the possibility of purchasing whole animals. Most people (including me!) may not have the room to purchase and store an entire cow or other large animal. I would suggest starting with smaller animals like duck, turkey, chicken, pheasant, rabbit, and fish.

The most cost-effective way to use the animal is to **break it down yourself.** Breaking down a chicken, or any other small animal, requires skill and a sharp knife. If you have not deboned an animal before, I would highly recommend that you take a class at a local cooking school or simply watch it being done online or in a video. Thanks to the internet, there are literally hundreds of experts/chefs teaching viewers how to safely and efficiently break down an animal. Including me! There is a video on my website (Andreabeaman.com/health) called ***Breaking Down the Bird***, that walks you through this process.

If you do *not* have the time or desire to sit and watch a video or learn a new skill, don't sweat it. Purchase a naturally raised animal at the local market and ask the butcher or fishmonger to break it down for you. It may cost a little extra to have them do the work, but you will still come out ahead.

Tell the butcher or fishmonger you want ALL (or most) of the pieces: bones, fat, skin, feet, carcass, and major internal organs (liver, heart, neck, and giblets). For larger animals like lamb, pig, and cow, I would suggest purchasing smaller pieces, or bones and feet only, instead of the entire animal. Try marrow bones, stock bones, knuckle bones, feet, necks, shanks, or oxtail. Most markets sell these animal parts at little cost.

Another way to get your hands on some nourishing bones is to save them from food you are already consuming. How many of us sit down to meals, devour the flesh, and discard the bones? I know I used to – before I became stock savvy. Each time you dine out in a restaurant or purchase cooked meat on the bone (osso bucco, braised lamb shank, chicken legs or wings, roasted duck, rotisserie chicken, and fried whole fish), there lies an opportunity to acquire bones. Don't be shy; ask for a doggie bag. You've paid for the meal (including the bones), and you can certainly take them with you. If you feel embarrassed, tell the server the bones are for your precious little doggie Fido or Twinkles the cat.

You can safely store bones in the freezer in a freezer-safe bag or container for a few months, and use them when you have accumulated enough (1 to 3 pounds). The more bones and other scraps you gather, the richer the stock. Make no bones about it, homemade stock is good nutrition.

The stock recipes in this chapter are basic and easy. You can also roast bones prior to boiling to acquire more depth of flavor. I've included a recipe for vegetable stock because, although vegetable stocks may not contain the protein, collagen, and amino acid profile of bone stock, they do contain vitamins and minerals and can enhance the flavor of food. I've also included a slow cooker version of stock.

It's time to call a meeting with the shareholders of your company (family members) and inform them their stock is about to increase!

BASIC CHICKEN STOCK

Bones of one free-range pastured chicken (carcass, neck, wingtips, feet, etc.), about 1 to 2 pounds
6 to 7 quarts water
2 onions, peeled and quartered
3 carrots, chopped
3 to 4 sprigs fresh thyme or 1 teaspoon dried
1/4 bunch fresh parsley with stems
1 tablespoon whole peppercorns

Procedure:

1. Bring bones and water to a boil in an 8-quart pot.
2. Skim off foam or scum that initially rises to the top of the pot and discard.
3. Add onions, carrots, thyme, parsley, and peppercorns.
4. Return to a boil.
5. Reduce heat and simmer, covered.
6. Cook for 4 to 10 hours. The longer you cook stock, the more concentrated it becomes.
7. Strain liquid, and discard bones and vegetables.
8. Place stock in the refrigerator and let fat congeal overnight.
9. Skim off the fat (chicken fat is called schmaltz). You can either discard the fat or use it for frying. Saturated animal fats have a higher smoke point than vegetable, nut, and seed oils, and don't oxidize as easily.
10. Pour defatted stock into freezer-safe containers, but do NOT fill to the top -- stock expands as it freezes.
11. Freeze stock for up to 3 months.

DUCK STOCK

The bones of one whole free-range, pastured duck (carcass, neck, wingtips, etc.), about 1 pound
6 quarts water
1 tablespoon butter (optional)
1 cup red wine
2 onions, peeled and quartered
3 carrots, chopped
2 garlic cloves
6 to 8 sprigs fresh thyme or 1 teaspoon dried
1/4 bunch fresh parsley
1 tablespoon whole peppercorns
1 bay leaf

Procedure:

1. Bring bones and water to a boil in an 8-quart pot.
2. Skim off foam or scum that rises to the top and discard.
3. Add butter, wine, onions, carrots, garlic, thyme, parsley, peppercorns and bay leaf.
4. Return to a boil.
5. Reduce heat; cover and simmer 6 to 12 hours. The longer you cook stock, the more concentrated it becomes.
6. Strain liquid, and discard bones and vegetables.
7. Place stock in the refrigerator and let fat congeal overnight.
8. Skim off fat -- discard the fat or use it for frying. Saturated animal fat has a high smoke point and is best for frying and baking.
9. Pour defatted stock into freezer-safe containers, but do NOT fill to the top - stock expands as it freezes.

TURKEY STOCK

The bones of one free-range, pastured turkey (carcass, neck, wings, etc.), about 2 pounds
6 to 7 quarts water
2 onions, peeled and quartered
2 celery stalks, chopped
3 carrots, chopped
3 to 4 sprigs fresh thyme or 1 teaspoon dried
1/4 bunch fresh parsley
2 to 3 fresh sage leaves or ½ teaspoon dried
1 tablespoon whole peppercorns

Procedure:

1. Bring bones and water to a boil in an 8-quart pot.
2. Skim off foam or scum that rises to the top and discard.
3. Add onions, celery, carrots, thyme, parsley, sage, and peppercorns.
4. Return to a boil.
5. Reduce heat and simmer, covered, for 6 to 12 hours.
6. Strain liquid, and discard bones and vegetables.
7. Place liquid in the refrigerator and let fat congeal overnight.
8. Skim off fat – you can either discard the fat or use it for frying.
9. Pour defatted stock into freezer-safe containers, but do NOT fill to the top – stock expands when it freezes.
10. You can safely store stock in the freezer for up to 3 months.

BEEF STOCK

2 pounds knuckles, marrow, shank, or other bones
6 to 7 quarts water
2 onions, peeled and quartered
3 carrots, chopped
2 celery stalks, chopped
2 garlic cloves, peeled
1/4 bunch fresh parsley
2 bay leaves
1 tablespoon whole peppercorns

Procedure:

1. Bring bones and water to a boil in an 8-quart pot.
2. Skim off foam or scum that rises to the top and discard.
3. Add onions, carrots, celery, garlic, parsley, bay leaves, and peppercorns.
4. Bring back up to a boil, then reduce heat, and simmer covered, 6 to 10 hours.
5. Strain liquid, and discard bones and vegetables.
6. Place stock in the refrigerator and let fat congeal overnight.
7. Skim off fat (beef fat is called tallow) – you can either discard the fat or use it for frying. Tallow, which is a saturated fat, has a high smoke point and doesn't oxidize easily.
8. Pour stock into freezer-safe containers, but do NOT fill to the top – stock expands as it freezes.
9. You can freeze stock for up to 3 months.

BASIC VEGETABLE STOCK

1 tablespoon olive oil
2 large onions, peeled and quartered
3 carrots, chopped
2 stalks celery and leaves
1 leek, cleaned and sliced (both white and green parts)
2 to 3 cloves garlic, peeled
½ bunch fresh parsley
5 to 6 thyme sprigs
2 bay leaves
1 teaspoon sea salt
6 to 7 quarts water

Procedure:

1. Heat the oil in an 8-quart pot over medium high heat.
2. Add onions, carrots, celery, leeks, and garlic.
3. Cook until the vegetables are lightly browned.
4. Add herbs, salt, and water; bring to a boil.
5. Cover and simmer on low heat for 1 or 2 hours.
6. Strain and use, or cool and store in the freezer.
7. If freezing stock, leave 1 to 2 inches of empty space inside the container for expansion as the stock freezes.

SLOW COOKER STOCK

If you are nervous about leaving an unattended pot of food cooking on top of your stove for many hours, purchase a slow cooker. You can make any of the stock recipes in a slow cooker by making a few simple adjustments. I've used a simple chicken stock as an example.

BASIC CHICKEN STOCK *(can use any stock recipe)*

The bones of one whole free-range, pastured chicken (carcass, neck, wingtips, etc.), about 1 or 2 pounds
4 to 5 quarts water (depending on the size of your slow cooker)
1 onion, peeled and quartered
2 carrots, chopped
3 to 4 sprigs fresh thyme or 1 teaspoon dried
1/4 bunch fresh parsley
½ tablespoon whole peppercorns

Procedure:

1. Bring bones and water to a boil in a large pot.
2. Skim off foam or scum that rises to the top and discard.
3. Add onions, carrots, thyme, parsley, and peppercorns; return to a boil.
4. Remove from heat and pour the contents of the stockpot into a slow cooker.
5. Set the timer for 10 to 12 hours on low heat setting, and cover.
6. After the slow cooker shuts off, strain liquid and discard bones and vegetables.

Chapter 9

MEALS THAT WORK!

Many folks dread stepping into the kitchen. They envision being shackled to the stove slaving over fiery burners all day, all night….oh the horror! Cast those fears aside -- there are easy ways to save time in the kitchen. It is a misconception that healthful homemade food takes an endless amount of time to prepare. It doesn't. Making meals that work just takes a little advance menu planning, and I can show you how to do it. I'll also help you save money by teaching you how to make the most of your recent wholesome purchases.

When I first took on the task of self-care, I also worked full time at MTV Networks. My hours usually were 9 am to 6 pm. By the time I arrived home at night, it was 7 pm or later. I needed to figure out time-saving tips so I wouldn't spend the night boiling and toiling away in the kitchen.

Preparing one main meal and utilizing the leftovers in the days that followed helped me reduce kitchen time, save gobs of money, and create many healthful homemade meals in the process. If you can find the time to allot a couple of hours once or twice per week to cooking a main meal, you will have a variety of delicious foods available that can nourish and support your beautiful body.

If a couple of hours per week are too much of a burden, don't sweat it. In my "Lifestyle Strategies for the Healthy and Fabulous!" chapter, I will teach you how to make wise choices when dining out -- no cooking, just ordering.

When it comes to food preparation, pick a time and day when you can create the space and get into the kitchen without major distractions. Remember, this is about setting aside the time for two of the most traditional and fundamental functions of living: cooking and eating. Turn off the television (unless you're watching me hosting one of my healthful cooking shows). It's time to get reconnected with your own life. Creating a lifestyle that promotes vibrant health can be easy once you learn how to replace non-action time, like watching television, with action time devoted to home cooking.

Freeing up time and space to nourish our bodies becomes simple when we recognize old habits that may no longer serve us, and by being open and willing to build new enjoyable routines. Just as poor habits are created over time, better lifestyle habits can be created, too. Change doesn't happen overnight; it's a process that takes time. And, you are worth all the time and energy you invest in any act of self-care.

In the pages that follow, I will recommend various menu ideas and tell you how to incorporate leftovers into new and exciting dishes. From each of these menus, you can prepare one, two, or three *leftover* meals – whatever you have the capacity to take on.

Patience and persistence is imperative when you are learning a new habit. Think about it… how many of us would be habitual smokers if we had put down the cigarettes and not picked them up again and again? Pick up this recipe book and cook meals again and again and eventually you can create a *health-promoting* habit.

Experiment with the menus that call most strongly to your body. Override any "thoughts" about what you are supposed to eat, and let your body speak to you. Whether it is asking for beans, grains, noodles, turkey, chicken, fish, beef, or bone stocks, your body is brilliant and will guide you to eat exactly what you need. Your body is your own personal laboratory and the kitchen is where you can experiment with the foods that can make you feel healthy and strong.

One of the reasons animals in the wild remain relatively healthy and strong is because they haven't read any diet books recommending specific amounts of fat, carbohydrates, protein, vegetables and fruits to eat. Their bodies simply say, "Eat that grass, eat that deer, eat that bug, eat the honey, eat those berries, but do NOT eat the brightly colored frogs." And, they listen. If they don't follow their instincts… it's sayonara, baby!

I want to emphasize again that you do *not* have to prepare everything on the menus in the following pages. That may be overwhelming, especially if you are just getting started. I would suggest cooking any of the main meals and utilizing the leftovers to create *one* new dish the following day or the day after that, or anytime during the week when your schedule permits. Kept in airtight containers, leftovers can safely be used four to five days after their initial cooking.

When it comes to using leftovers, let your senses guide you. Open a container of food and take a sniff. If your nose scrunches up, your body recoils, and your arms forcefully shove the offending food as far away from your face as humanly possible…DO NOT EAT IT! Your nose knows. And, if you open a container of food and observe green fuzzy mold growing on the top (and it's not blue cheese), toss it out and send it back to the universe via the garbage!

Menu planning always begins with one main meal. For example, in one of my recent cooking classes I prepared:

Black-Eyed Peas with Chorizo (spicy pork sausage)
Basic Brown Rice
Braised Red Cabbage and Kale
Winter Cobbler

This meal took approximately 1½ hours from start to finish. It provided many opportunities to transform leftovers into other scrumptious dishes. On the following page is the main meal plus possible leftovers:

MENU #1

	Main Meal	Leftovers	Leftovers
Breakfast		Savory Rice & Oats Porridge	Warm Winter Cobbler and Tea
Lunch		Black-Eyed Peas with Braised Red Cabbage and Kale Wrap	
Dinner	Black-Eyed Peas with Chorizo Basic Brown Rice Braised Red Cabbage and Kale Winter Cobbler	Quick-Cooking Fried Rice	Black-Eyed Pea Soup with Whole Grain Bread

1. The main meal is prepared.
2. A portion of the leftover rice can be used to prepare a simple Savory Rice & Oats Porridge the following morning.
3. Leftover Black-Eyed Peas with Chorizo can be combined with Braised Red Cabbage and Kale, and wrapped in a whole grain burrito for lunch.

4. Quick-Cooking Fried Rice can be prepared for dinner using leftover rice.
5. If there happens to be any Winter Cobbler left over (highly unlikely), warm it up and have it for breakfast one morning. Yes, that's right, dessert for breakfast. The ingredients are fruit, rolled oats, and maple syrup for gosh sakes. If we can swallow stuff like Fruity Pebbles and Cocoa Puffs we can certainly eat leftover Winter Cobbler!
6. Finally, a Black-Eyed Pea Soup with whole grain bread could be prepared for another delicious dinner.

Most "leftover" dishes take anywhere from five to thirty minutes to prepare. Keep in mind, if you order Chinese takeout, pizza, or other food, it can take anywhere from thirty to forty minutes (or more) for the delivery to arrive. In that same amount of time (or less), you could prepare a meal loaded with nutrients and made with love.

Recipes follow directly after each menu plan. You do *not* have to create all the meals and menus exactly the way they are listed. Each recipe can also be used as a "stand-alone" dish and prepared whenever you want. Keep in mind, the larger the quantity of "main meal" you prepare, the more opportunity for leftovers. If you want to experiment with more leftovers, increase the quantity of the main meal.

There are seven full menus with many scrumptious options to choose from. You won't have to worry about getting hungry or growing bored with your food. I've already demonstrated Menu Plan #1; the recipes can be found in the pages that follow.

Below are six more menus, with their leftover possibilities, to give you an idea of what's cooking in this chapter:

Menu #2 (pg. 122)

Sesame-Crusted Sole

Simple Soba Noodles

Sautéed Bok Choy & Carrots

Soba Noodle Stir-Fry

Five-Minute Miso Soup

Menu #3 (pg. 130)

Baked Chicken & Rosemary-Roasted Potatoes

Simple Sautéed Carrots and Broccoli

Chicken Liver Pâté

Cheese and Veggie Omelet with Homey Home Fries

Quick-Cooking Chicken Cacciatore

Whole Grain Herbed Garlic Bread

Curried Chicken Salad

White Bean and Kale Soup with Crispy Garlic Croutons

Menu #4 (pg. 143)

Lentils with Sautéed Leeks, Spinach, and Sausage

Simple Brown Basmati Rice

Steamed Winter Vegetables with Toasted Walnuts and Cranberry Dressing

Lentil and Vegetable Wrap

Stir-Fried Shrimp, Rice, and Vegetables

Silky Lentil Soup

Creamy Coconut Rice Pudding

<u>Menu #5 (pg. 154)</u>

Basic Black Beans

Polenta with Sautéed Shitake Mushrooms and Turkey Sausage

Fried Polenta Squares

Seasonal Bean Salad in Lettuce Cups

Spicy Black Bean Soup with Polenta Croutons

<u>Menu #6 (pg. 161)</u>

Roasted Turkey with Herbed Gravy

Whole Grain Couscous with Dried Cranberries

Savory Couscous Porridge

Sautéed Collard Greens with Garlic

Turkey Chowder

Turkey and Pasta Salad

Hot Opened Turkey Sandwich with Herbed Gravy

<u>Menu 7 (pg. 172)</u>

Tahini Noodles & Braised Duck

Rendered Duck Fat

Hearty Roasted Winter Roots

Sautéed Brussels Sprouts with Cranberries & Toasted Almonds

Savory Shitake Mushroom Soup

Pan-Seared Duck Breast & Chinese Cabbage Salad with Crunchy Cracklins

Duck Liver Pâté

Caramelized Onion Soup

Choose one of these many menu plans and go for it. Prepare one new plan per week. And, remember to have fun with your food!

BLACK-EYED PEAS WITH CHORIZO

1½ cups dried black-eyed peas, soaked in water to cover for 6 to 8 hours

3 cups water

2 bay leaves

1½ teaspoons sea salt, divided

1½ tablespoons olive oil

2 onions, peeled and diced

5 garlic cloves, peeled and minced

2 cups chicken stock (or liquid from cooked black-eyed peas)

1 tablespoon fresh oregano or 1 teaspoon dried

3 to 4 ounces dried chorizo sausage, diced

Freshly ground black pepper

1 tablespoon minced fresh parsley

Preparation:

1. Drain black-eyed peas and discard soaking water.
2. In a large pot, bring 3 cups fresh water and soaked peas to a boil.
3. Skim and discard foam that rises to the top.
4. Add bay leaves. Reduce heat and simmer, covered, for one hour.
5. Add 1 teaspoon sea salt and continue cooking 15 to 20 minutes or until beans soften. Remove and discard bay leaves.
6. In a deep frying pan, heat oil, and sauté onion and garlic 2 to 3 minutes.
7. Add black-eyed peas, stock, oregano, and chorizo.
8. Season the dish with remaining 1/2 teaspoon sea salt and black pepper to taste.
9. Cover and cook on medium-low heat for 10 to 12 minutes.
10. Garnish with fresh parsley.

If strapped for time, canned beans can be used in any recipe. Always remember to rinse canned beans as they contain complex sugars, arrinose and stachyose, that contribute to gas and bloating. Soaking dried beans begins the breakdown of those sugars. If they are not broken down before you eat them, they will be consumed by bacteria in the digestive tract, leading to the release of methane as a byproduct, aka… gas!

Canned beans may contribute to gas and bloating because those complex sugars remain inside the can after the canning process. When rinsing canned beans you may notice a mysterious foam. That's what I call the "fart foam." Just rinse it off and send it down the drain to wash away this potential odorous dilemma.

Variation: If using canned beans for this recipe, begin preparation at step 6. There is no need to soak and cook canned beans because they are already cooked.

BASIC BROWN RICE

2 cups short grain brown rice, soaked in water for 6 to 8 hours (or overnight)
3¾ cups water
2 pinches sea salt

Preparation:

1. Discard rice soaking water
2. In a pot, bring rice and water to a boil
3. Add sea salt
4. Cover, reduce heat, and simmer 45 minutes

SAVORY RICE & OATS PORRIDGE

1 cup leftover or cooked rice
3 tablespoons rolled oats
2 tablespoons butter
2 cups water
¼ cup diced dried apricots
1 dash nutmeg
1/3 cup walnuts, roasted and chopped
¼ cup almond or other milk

Preparation:

1. In a medium pot, bring rice, oats, butter, water, apricots, and nutmeg to a boil.
2. Cover, reduce heat to low, and simmer for 7 to 9 minutes.
3. Put into a bowl and top with roasted walnuts and a splash of milk.

BRAISED RED CABBAGE AND KALE

1 onion, peeled and sliced in thin crescents
1 tablespoon olive oil or other fat (chicken, duck)*
¼ head red or green cabbage, shredded
2 or 3 kale leaves, thinly sliced
1 green apple, cut in matchsticks
½ teaspoon sea salt
1 tablespoon honey
2 tablespoons apple cider vinegar
½ cup water or chicken stock

Preparation:

1. In a skillet, over medium heat, sauté onion in olive oil for 1 to 2 minutes.
2. Add cabbage, kale, and green apple. Sauté 2 to 3 minutes.
3. Add sea salt, honey, vinegar, and water.
4. Cover and cook on medium-low heat for 25 to 30 minutes.

*You will learn how to render duck and chicken fats in Menu #7. Duck fat, like all poultry fats, is mainly monounsaturated and is low in polyunsaturated fat, which makes it a good fat for cooking and frying.[35]

---

[35] Fat, An Appreciation of a Misunderstood Ingredient, Jennifer McLagan, Ten Speed Press, 2008, p. 124

WINTER COBBLER

Filling:

3 pears, cored and diced
3 apples, cored and diced
¼ cup dried cranberries
½ cup apple juice
1 teaspoon ginger juice (grate ginger, squeezed, pulp discarded)
½ teaspoon ground cinnamon
¼ teaspoon ground cloves
2 tablespoons whole grain pastry flour
1/8 teaspoon sea salt

Topping:

¾ cup whole grain pastry flour
½ cup rolled oats
1/3 cup granulated maple sugar or other sugar
½ teaspoon baking powder
¼ teaspoon sea salt
3 to 4 tablespoons butter, softened

Preparation:

1. Preheat oven to 375° F.
2. Put diced pears, apples, and dried cranberries into a 9-inch square casserole or baking dish.
3. In a small bowl, whisk together apple juice, ginger juice, cinnamon, cloves, flour, and salt.
4. Pour mixture onto fruit and toss to coat thoroughly.
5. In a separate bowl, combine flour, oats, maple sugar, baking powder and salt.

6. Work softened butter into the flour until you have a crumbly mixture.
7. Sprinkle crumbles on top of fruit.
8. Cover and bake 25 to 30 minutes.
9. Uncover and continue baking 35 minutes or until crumble topping is lightly browned and filling is bubbling to the surface.

BLACK-EYED PEA SOUP

1 cup dried black-eyed peas, soaked in water for 8 hours + 3 additional cups water
OR 2 cups leftover Black-Eyed Peas and Chorizo
OR 2 (15-ounce) cans black-eyed peas, rinsed and drained
1 tablespoon olive oil
1 onion, peeled and diced
2 celery stalks, diced
3 carrots, diced
2 garlic cloves, peeled and minced
1 teaspoon sea salt
4 cups chicken stock
1 tablespoon fresh thyme or 1 teaspoon dried
Freshly ground black pepper

Preparation from scratch:

1. If using dried peas, discard soaking water from the peas.
2. In a pot, bring 3 cups fresh water and peas to a boil. Skim and discard foam that rises to the top.
3. Cover, reduce heat, and simmer 1 hour.
4. If using leftover or canned peas, skip Step #1 thru #3 and add the peas in Step #6.
5. In a separate pan, heat olive oil and sauté onions, celery, carrots, and garlic.
6. Add black-eyed peas, salt, chicken stock, and thyme, and pepper to taste.
7. Bring back up to a boil, then reduce heat to medium. Cook covered 20 to 25 minutes or until vegetables soften.

SAUTÉED BLACK-EYED PEAS AND VEGETABLE WRAP

1 tablespoon olive oil or other fat* (chicken fat, duck fat)

½ cup cooked black-eyed peas

½ cup cooked braised cabbage and kale

Whole Grain Burrito Wraps

Preparation:

1. In a skillet, heat black-eyed peas and cabbage in olive oil.
2. In a separate frying pan, over low heat, warm the burrito wrap.
3. Lay warmed wrap on a flat surface and fill with bean and cabbage mixture.
4. Roll up and enjoy!

QUICK-COOKING FRIED RICE

2 tablespoons peanut oil, divided

2 eggs, beaten

1 onion, peeled and diced

2 garlic cloves, peeled and minced

3 to 4 button mushrooms, thinly sliced

1/2 teaspoon sea salt

1 cup cooked or leftover brown rice

1 stalk broccoli, florets and stem (dice the stem)

1 tablespoon toasted sesame oil

2 tablespoons shoyu

1 tablespoon mirin*

¼ to 1/3 cup water (or chicken stock)

2 scallions, minced

Preparation:

1. In a skillet, heat 1 tablespoon oil and scramble the eggs, breaking them into small pieces.
2. Remove eggs from the skillet and set aside.
3. Add remaining 1 tablespoon oil, and sauté onions and garlic 1 to 2 minutes.
4. Add mushrooms and salt, and sauté 1 to 2 minutes.
5. Add brown rice and broccoli to the skillet.
6. Combine toasted sesame oil, shoyu, mirin, and water, and add to the skillet.
7. Cover and cook on medium heat 5 to 7 minutes, or until broccoli is tender.

8. Return cooked scrambled egg pieces to the pan and toss with vegetables and rice.
9. Garnish with minced scallions.

Mirin is sweet rice cooking wine – you can substitute maple syrup or other liquid sweetener in this recipe or omit it entirely.

Menu Plan #2

	Main Meal	Leftovers	Leftovers
Breakfast		Make a nourishing fish stock with the bones (and head)	Five-Minute Miso Soup
Lunch			
Dinner	Sesame-Crusted Sole (if using whole fish, reserve the bones and head for stock) Simple Soba Noodles Sautéed Bok Choy & Carrots	Soba Noodle Stir-Fry	

This simple menu is designed for folks who have very limited time to cook, but still want to enjoy delicious and nutritious meals. The main meal can be prepared and ready to eat in 15 to 20 minutes.

1. Sesame-Crusted Sole, Simple Soba Noodles, and Sautéed Bok Choy & Carrots are the main meal.
2. Prepare a nourishing fish stock. All the ingredients can be put on the stove and be left cooking all day.

3. Enjoy a Soba Noodle Stir-Fry the following night for dinner.
4. A Five-Minute Miso Soup can easily be prepared in the morning for breakfast. That is probably less time than waiting on line at the local Starbucks for a cup of coffee and a darn cinnamon roll!

SESAME-CRUSTED SOLE

1 tablespoon maple syrup
½ cup water
2 tablespoons shoyu (naturally fermented soy sauce)
2 garlic cloves, peeled and minced
1-inch piece fresh ginger, peeled and minced
12 to 16 ounces lemon sole, fluke, or flounder fillets (or two whole fish filleted – reserve the bones to make fish stock)
4 tablespoons black sesame seeds
2 tablespoons tan sesame seeds
1/3 cup flour
Sea salt
2 to 3 tablespoons coconut oil

Preparation:

1. Combine maple syrup, water, shoyu, garlic, and ginger in a bowl.
2. Marinate fish in the mixture 15 to 20 minutes on the counter or overnight, covered, in the refrigerator.
3. In a small bowl, combine black and tan sesame seeds, flour, and a couple pinches of salt.
4. Remove fish from marinade (do not discard) and coat fish with flour mixture.
5. Heat oil in a pan over medium-high heat.
6. Pan sear fish fillets 2 minutes on each side.
7. In a small saucepot, bring reserved marinade to a boil over high heat. Cook, uncovered, until reduced by two thirds.
8. To serve, drizzle marinade reduction on top of fish.
9. Sit down.

10. Take a deep breath and relax.
11. Say grace or be thankful for something (the food you are about to eat, the home chef that prepared it, and the charismatic cookbook author that showed you how to do it).
12. Enjoy!

SIMPLE SOBA NOODLES

Water
8 ounces soba noodles
3 tablespoons toasted sesame oil
2 tablespoons shoyu
1½ tablespoons brown rice vinegar
½ tablespoon black or tan sesame seeds, toasted
1 scallion, minced
½ tsp. dulse flakes

Preparation:

1. Bring water to a boil in a saucepot.
2. Add noodles and cook according to package directions (7 to 10 minutes).
3. In a small bowl, whisk sesame oil, shoyu, and rice vinegar to make dressing.
4. Drain noodles and combine with dressing and toasted sesame seeds.
5. Garnish with minced scallions and dulse flakes.

SAUTÉED BOK CHOY & CARROTS

3 carrots, thinly cut on the diagonal

1/4 cup water

3 to 4 bok choy leaves, in bite-size pieces

1 teaspoon toasted sesame oil

1 teaspoon shoyu

Preparation:

1. In a skillet, over high heat, cook carrots in the water for 2 to 3 minutes.
2. Add bok choy, cover, and steam 1 to 2 minutes.
3. Drizzle with sesame oil and shoyu.
4. Cook an additional 2 to 3 minutes, or until vegetables are wilted.

SOBA NOODLE STIR-FRY

2 tablespoons peanut oil, divided

2 eggs, beaten

1 onion, peeled and diced

2 garlic cloves, peeled and minced

1 teaspoon ginger, peeled and minced

3 to 4 mushrooms, thinly sliced

1/2 teaspoon sea salt

1 to 1½ cups cooked soba or other noodles

1 stalk broccoli, florets and stem (dice the stem)

1 tablespoon toasted sesame oil

2 tablespoons shoyu

1 tablespoon mirin rice cooking wine (or other sweetener)

1/3 cup water

2 scallions, minced

1 tablespoon cilantro, minced

½ sheet toasted nori sea vegetable, cut in thin strips

Preparation:

1. In a frying pan, heat 1 tablespoon peanut oil and scramble the eggs, breaking them into small pieces.
2. Remove eggs from the pan.
3. Add remaining 1 tablespoon peanut oil to the pan, and sauté onions, garlic, and ginger 1 to 2 minutes.
4. Add mushrooms and salt and sauté for 1 to 2 minutes.
5. Add noodles and broccoli to the pan.
6. In a small bowl, combine toasted sesame oil, shoyu, mirin, and water; add to the pan.
7. Cover and cook on medium heat 5 to 7 minutes, or until broccoli is tender.
8. Return cooked egg pieces to the pan and toss with vegetables and noodles.
9. Garnish with minced scallions, cilantro and strips of nori.

FIVE-MINUTE MISO SOUP

4 cups water or fish stock

1 teaspoon ginger, minced

1-inch piece wakame sea vegetable

2 carrots, thinly cut diagonally

4 to 6 ounces fish or tofu, in one-inch cubes

1 to 2 bok choy leaves, in bite-size pieces

3 tablespoons sweet/light miso

Leftover noodles or other cooked grain

2 scallions, minced

Preparation:

1. In a saucepot, bring water, ginger, wakame, and carrots to a boil.
2. Reduce heat to medium.
3. Add fish and bok choy to the soup and cook 2 to -3 minutes.
4. Dilute miso in a small amount of water and add to soup.
5. Simmer 2 to 3 minutes.
6. Put leftover noodles or grain in the bottom of a soup bowl.
7. Ladle soup on top of noodles and garnish with minced scallions.

Menu Plan #3 (Weekend Menu)

	Main Meal	Leftovers	Leftovers
Brunch		Cheese and Veggie Omelet Homey Home Fries Make Chicken Stock (recipe in the stock chapter)	Sleep late, rest, snuggle under the covers with your sweetheart Go out for a fun brunch at a local Mom and Pop joint
Snack		Chicken Liver Pâté on Whole Grain Crackers	Curried Chicken Salad
Dinner	Baked Chicken & Rosemary-Roasted Potatoes Simple Sautéed Carrots and Broccoli	Quick-Cooking Chicken Cacciatore Whole Grain Herbed Garlic Bread	White Bean and Kale Soup with Crispy Garlic Croutons

1. Baked Chicken & Rosemary-Roasted Vegetables, and Simple Sautéed Carrots and Broccoli are the main meal.
2. The leftover potatoes can be used for Homey Home Fries, and an omelet can be made with the leftover sautéed veggies.

3. If you are lucky enough to get the chicken livers with your chicken (very rare these days), make a nourishing pâté, rich in vitamins A, D, and B12, plus iron.
4. The chicken carcass can be used to make a nourishing health-supportive bone stock.
5. Leftover chicken wings and drumsticks are delicious in an easy chicken cacciatore dish.
6. On Saturday or Sunday morning, stay in bed, relax, and chill out. For real! Monday begins the work week... again. Make sure you are well rested and refreshed. The way our society is set up, there is a tendency to work, work, work, nonstop, with few rejuvenation periods, if any. I recall some important info from a religious instruction class:

"And on the seventh day God ended his work which he had made; and he rested on the seventh day from all his work which he had made."[36]

For the ladies reading this please substitute "Goddess" for "God" and "she" for "he." It's imperative we incorporate rest periods into our life. If we don't find the time to rest, the universe will force *rest* upon us in the form of an achy flu or other bug that keeps us in bed for a couple of days, or worse yet, a debilitating disease that can keep us down for a longer period of time. Trust me, if the great "creator of all things" can rest on the seventh day, so can you. After all, you are the creator of your life. Okay.... enough proselytizing! Back to the menu:

7. Prepare Curried Chicken Salad with leftover roasted chicken.

[36] http://bible.cc/genesis/2-2.htm

8. Make White Bean and Kale Soup with Crispy Garlic Croutons with half the chicken stock (freeze the other half for later use).
9. Use leftover garlic bread to make croutons for soup.

BAKED CHICKEN & ROSEMARY-ROASTED POTATOES

1 whole pastured or free-range chicken
2 tablespoons butter, softened (optional)
Sea salt
Freshly ground black pepper
2 onions, peeled and chopped
6 to 8 red or new potatoes, quartered
1 teaspoon dried rosemary
1 tablespoon olive oil or schmaltz (chicken fat)

Preparation:

1. Preheat oven to 350° F.
2. Rinse chicken under running water and pat dry.
3. Rub butter under chicken skin (optional).
4. Season the outside of the chicken with salt and pepper to taste.
5. Place the chicken in a baking pan.
6. In a mixing bowl combine onions, potatoes, rosemary, and olive oil; season with salt and pepper to taste.
7. Place onions and potatoes in the baking pan around the chicken.
8. Cover and bake approximately 12 to 15 minutes per pound of chicken.
9. Uncover the chicken two-thirds of the way through the cooking, crank up the heat to 425° F, and baste with juices from the bottom of the pan to ensure the skin becomes crispy, brown, and delicious!

SIMPLE SAUTÉED CARROTS AND BROCCOLI

½ cup water or chicken stock
2 to 3 carrots, cut ½-inch thick on the diagonal
Sea salt
1 head broccoli, florets chopped and stem diced
1 tablespoon grass-fed butter
1 garlic clove, peeled and minced

Preparation:

1. Put water and carrots into a frying pan with a pinch of sea salt and cook 1 to 2 minutes on medium-high heat.
2. Add broccoli stems to the pan and cook 1 minute.
3. Add broccoli florets, butter, garlic, and another pinch of sea salt and cook 3 to 5 minutes.

CHICKEN LIVER PÂTÉ

½ cup water or chicken stock

2 or 3 pastured, free-range chicken livers (I save my chicken livers in the freezer until I have enough to make pâté)

2 shallots, peeled and diced or 2 tablespoons chopped onion

1 garlic clove, peeled and minced

1 bay leaf

1 teaspoon fresh thyme or ½ teaspoon dried

2 to 3 tablespoons softened butter, divided

2 tablespoons white wine OR 2 teaspoons brandy

Sea salt

Freshly ground black pepper

Whole grain rye crackers

Preparation:

1. Cut chicken livers in half and clean (remove excess fat and blood).
2. In a small saucepan, heat the chicken stock, chicken livers, shallots, garlic, bay leaf, thyme, 1 tablespoon butter, and wine.
3. Bring to a boil, reduce heat and simmer 2 to 3 minutes.
4. Add salt and pepper to taste, and cook 1 minute more.
5. Remove and discard bay leaf.
6. With a slotted spoon, separate chicken livers, shallots, and garlic from any liquid that may remain in the saucepan, and put into a food processor or blender with remaining 2 tablespoons softened butter.
7. Puree until smooth and creamy (can add liquid from the cooking pan to achieve a creamier consistency).
8. Put into a small container or jar and refrigerate until jelled.
9. Smear on whole grain rye crackers or toast.

CHEESE AND VEGGIE OMELET

1 tablespoon grass-fed butter or olive oil

4 eggs (or 2 eggs per person)

¼ cup raw milk cheddar cheese, grated

1 cup leftover or steamed vegetables (broccoli, carrots), finely diced

Sea salt

Freshly ground black pepper

Preparation:

1. Melt butter in a frying pan over low heat.
2. Beat eggs in a bowl and pour into the pan.
3. Roll eggs around the pan to distribute evenly.
4. Let eggs firm up a little (eggs cook very quickly!).
5. Add grated cheese and veggies into the center of the eggs.
6. Season with salt and pepper to taste.
7. With a spatula, gently fold the outer edges of the eggs over the vegetables.
8. Slide omelet out of the pan and onto a plate.

HOMEY HOME FRIES

Potatoes any way, anyhow, any day of the week, always taste like comfort food. If you're craving "home" this may be a good way to get there.

2 tablespoons butter or schmaltz*
1 tablespoon olive oil
1 onion, peeled and diced
3 to 4 potatoes, cooked and diced
Sea salt
Freshly ground black pepper

Preparation:

1. Melt butter and olive oil in a frying pan over medium heat.
2. Add onion and cook 3 to 4 minutes or until translucent.
3. Add potatoes and salt and pepper to taste.
4. Continue cooking 7 to 10 minutes or until potatoes are lightly browned.

Schmaltz is chicken fat – you can acquire schmaltz by rendering excess fat from the chicken. Directions for rendering fat is in Menu # 7 (Duck menu).

QUICK-COOKING CHICKEN CACCIATORE

1 tablespoon olive oil
1 tablespoon grass-fed butter
1 large onion, cut into thick crescents
5 to 6 button or cremini mushrooms, thickly sliced
2 to 3 garlic cloves, peeled and diced
1 (15-ounce) can diced tomatoes with juice
1/3 cup water or chicken stock
1 teaspoon dried oregano or 1 tablespoon fresh
½ tablespoon dried basil or 1½ tablespoon fresh
12 ounces raw chicken breast, diced or any cooked chicken parts
½ teaspoon sea salt
Freshly ground black pepper

Preparation:

1. In a skillet, over medium heat, heat oil and butter. Sauté onion for 1 to 2 minutes.
2. Add mushrooms and garlic, and cook 2 to 3 minutes.
3. Add diced tomatoes, water, oregano, and basil.
4. If using raw diced chicken breast, add to the pan with salt and pepper to taste. Cook, covered, 5 to 7 minutes.
5. If using cooked chicken parts, add to the pan, season with salt and pepper to taste. Cook, covered 3 to 4 minutes.

WHOLE GRAIN HERBED GARLIC BREAD

Whole wheat baguette (or any other whole grain thin/long bread loaf)
2 tablespoons olive oil
2 tablespoons butter, softened
2 garlic cloves, peeled and minced
Mixed dried herbs (oregano, basil, rosemary, or marjoram)
Sea salt

Preparation:

1. Preheat oven to 375° F.
2. Cut baguette in half lengthwise.
3. In a small bowl, combine olive oil, butter, garlic, and one or two pinches of dried herb.
4. Brush or spoon the olive oil mixture onto the bread.
5. Season with sea salt to taste.
6. Wrap the bread with aluminum foil and bake 3 to 5 minutes.
7. Unwrap the bread (careful, it's hot!) and continue baking 5 to 7 minutes, or until lightly browned and crispy.

CURRIED CHICKEN SALAD

10 to 12 ounces poached or cooked chicken, diced
2 celery stalks, diced
1/4 cup minced cilantro
1 apple, cored and diced
1/4 cup extra virgin olive oil
2 tablespoons apple cider vinegar
2 to 3 tablespoons mayonnaise
1 1/2 teaspoons curry powder
1/2 teaspoon sea salt
Freshly ground black pepper

Preparation:

1. Combine chicken, celery, cilantro, and apple in a mixing bowl.
2. In a small bowl, whisk olive oil, vinegar, mayonnaise, curry powder, and salt.
3. Combine dressing with chicken mixture and toss to coat evenly.
4. Season with black pepper to taste; add more salt if needed.

WHITE BEAN AND KALE SOUP WITH CRISPY GARLIC CROUTONS

1 large onion, peeled and diced

3 garlic cloves, peeled and minced

1 tablespoon olive oil

2 to 3 kale leaves, cleaned and thinly sliced

4 cups chicken stock

1/4 teaspoon dried rosemary

1 teaspoon dried thyme

3 cups cooked cannelini beans or two (15-ounce) cans, rinsed

1 teaspoon sea salt

Freshly ground black pepper

Preparation:

1. Sauté onion and garlic in olive oil in a frying pan for 2 to 3 minutes.
2. Add kale and cook until wilted.
3. Add chicken stock, rosemary, and thyme.
4. For a creamier consistency, puree 1/2 the beans in a food processor or blender. Add all the beans to the pot.
5. Bring all ingredients to a boil.
6. Reduce heat to medium-low, cover, and cook 7 to 10 minutes.
7. Season with salt and pepper to taste.
8. Serve with Crispy Garlic Croutons (recipe on the following page).

CRISPY GARLIC CROUTONS

Leftover Whole Grain Herbed Garlic Bread or fresh whole grain baguette

Olive oil

2 garlic cloves, peeled and minced

Sea salt

Preparation:

1. Dice leftover garlic bread and bake at 350° F for 5 minutes or until crispy.
2. If using fresh bread (whole grain baguette), dice into cubes, season with olive oil, minced garlic, and sea salt, and place onto a baking tray.
3. Bake in the oven 7 to 10 minutes or until crispy.

Menu Plan #4

	Main Meal	Leftovers	Leftovers
Breakfast	Soak lentils Soak rice		
Lunch		Lentil and Vegetable Wrap	Take leftovers from the previous night's dinner for lunch
Dinner	Lentils with Sautéed Leeks, Spinach, and Sausage Simple Brown Basmati Rice Steamed Winter Vegetables with Toasted Walnuts and Cranberry Dressing	Stir-Fried Shrimp, Rice, and Vegetables	Silky Lentil Soup Creamy Coconut Rice Pudding

1. Soak rice and lentils in separate bowls.
2. Prepare Lentils with Sautéed Leeks, Spinach and Sausage, Simple Brown Basmati Rice and Steamed Winter Vegetables with Toasted Walnuts and Cranberry Dressing for dinner.

3. The following day, wrap leftover lentils and vegetables for lunch.
4. Prepare a simple Stir-Fried Shrimp and Vegetables for dinner.
5. Use leftover lentils to prepare Silky Lentil soup.
6. Leftover rice can be used to create Creamy Coconut Rice Pudding. Ooh la la!

LENTILS WITH SAUTÉED LEEKS, SPINACH, AND SAUSAGE

1 tablespoon olive oil
2 garlic cloves, peeled and minced
1 large leek, cleaned and chopped (both white and green parts)
½ bunch spinach, cleaned and chopped
1 tablespoon fresh thyme
1½ cups green, brown, or black lentils, soaked overnight in water to cover, drained
3½ cups chicken stock or water
2 bay leaves
2 to 3 sausage links (pork, chicken, or turkey), diced
½ teaspoon sea salt
2 tablespoons minced fresh parsley

Preparation:

1. In a large pot, heat oil and sauté garlic and leek for 1 to 2 minutes.
2. Add spinach and cook until wilted, or 2 to 3 minutes.
3. Add thyme, lentils (discard lentil soaking water), chicken stock, and bay leaves.
4. Bring to a boil; cover and simmer on low 45 minutes.
5. Add diced sausage and sea salt.
6. Taste and adjust seasoning.
7. Cook an additional 15 to 20 minutes.
8. Remove and discard bay leaves.
9. Serve garnished with minced parsley.

SIMPLE BROWN BASMATI RICE

2 cups long grain brown basmati rice, soaked in water to cover for 6 to 8 hours

3½ cups water

2 pinches sea salt

Preparation:

1. Drain rice and discard soaking water.
2. In a medium pot, bring rice and water to a boil.
3. Add salt.
4. Cover, reduce heat and simmer for 35 to 40 minutes.

STEAMED WINTER VEGETABLES WITH TOASTED WALNUTS AND CRANBERRY DRESSING

2 to 3 carrots, cut into ½-inch thick rounds or diagonals
Sea salt
1 bunch kale, cut into bite-size pieces
½ head cabbage, thinly sliced
1/3 cup roasted walnuts (see the following pages for directions on roasting and toasting nuts)
2 tablespoons dried cranberries

Preparation:

1. Put steamer basket into a pot with a few inches of water and turn heat up to high.
2. Add carrots and a pinch of sea salt.
3. Cover and steam 2 to 3 minutes.
4. Place kale and cabbage and another pinch sea salt on top of carrots and steam an additional 5 to 7 minutes, or until bright green and tender.
5. Transfer veggies to a large mixing bowl.
6. Toss steamed veggies with Cranberry Dressing and garnish with toasted walnuts and dried cranberries.

CRANBERRY DRESSING

1/3 cup walnut oil

2 tablespoons apple cider vinegar

2 tablespoons cranberry juice concentrate

1 to 2 tablespoons maple syrup

Sea salt and freshly ground black pepper

Preparation:

1. In a small bowl, combine oil, vinegar, cranberry juice concentrate, and maple syrup.
2. Add salt and pepper to taste.

ROASTING NUTS

To roast walnuts, or any other nut:

4. Preheat oven to 350° F.
5. Place raw nuts onto a baking sheet.
6. Roast in the oven, shaking the pan occasionally, for 8 to 10 minutes, or until lightly browned.

TOASTING NUTS

To toast nuts on top of the stove:

5. Heat a skillet over low heat.
6. Place raw nuts into the skillet without any oil.
7. Gently shake or move the nuts frequently to prevent them from burning.
8. The nuts will become lightly browned and release a "nutty fragrance" when they are done (approximately 10 to 12 minutes).

LENTIL AND VEGETABLE WRAP

½ cup leftover Lentils with Sautéed Leeks, Spinach, and Sausage or ½ cup canned lentils, rinsed and drained
1 tablespoon olive oil
½ cup steamed cabbage and kale
Sea salt
Whole grain burrito wraps
Cranberry Dressing

Preparation:

1. In a frying pan, heat leftover lentils and sausage (or rinsed canned lentils) in olive oil.
2. Place water and steamer basket into the bottom of a pot and bring to a boil.
3. Put cabbage and kale into the pot with a pinch of sea salt, cover, and steam 3 to 4 minutes or until bright green.
4. In a separate frying pan, over low heat, warm the burrito wrap.
5. Lay warmed wrap on a flat surface and fill with lentils and steamed vegetables.
6. Add 1 to 2 tablespoons of cranberry dressing.
7. Roll up and enjoy!

STIR-FRIED SHRIMP, RICE, AND VEGETABLES

1 tablespoon peanut oil

1 onion, peeled and diced

2 garlic cloves, peeled and minced

¼ teaspoon sea salt

2 stalks broccoli, florets and stem (dice the stem)

½ red pepper, seeded and cut into 1-inch pieces

6 to 8 ounces shrimp, or other protein (extra firm tofu, chicken, or beef), cubed

1 tablespoon toasted sesame oil

2 tablespoons shoyu (naturally fermented soy sauce)

1 tablespoon mirin rice wine (optional)

1/3 cup water or chicken stock

1/2 cup cooked brown rice per person

2 scallions, minced

Preparation:

1. In a frying pan, heat oil and sauté onion and garlic for 1 to 2 minutes.
2. Season with a pinch or two of sea salt.
3. Add broccoli florets and stems: cook 1 to 2 minutes.
4. Add red pepper and shrimp.
5. In a small bowl, combine the sesame oil, shoyu, mirin, and water and add to the pan.
6. Cover and cook on medium heat 3 to 5 minutes, or until broccoli is bright green.
7. Add rice to the pan, and toss with other ingredients.
8. Garnish with minced scallions.

SILKY LENTIL SOUP

1 tablespoon olive oil
1 onion, peeled and diced
2 garlic cloves, peeled and minced
2 carrots, diced
1 celery stalk, diced
1 tablespoon fresh thyme or 1 teaspoon dried
1 teaspoon sea salt
2 to 3 cups cooked lentils or two (15-ounce) cans lentils, rinsed and drained
4 cups chicken stock, beef stock, or water
¼ cup minced fresh parsley
Whole grain bread and grass-fed butter

Preparation:

1. Heat oil in a large frying pan over medium-high heat and sauté onions and garlic for 1 to 2 minutes.
2. Add carrots, celery, thyme, sea salt, lentils, and stock.
3. Bring to a boil, reduce heat to medium-low, and cook 15 to 20 minutes.
4. Remove approximately half of the lentils and vegetables and puree in a blender or food processor to give the soup a silky smooth consistency. Return to pot.
5. Garnish with fresh parsley.
6. Serve with a piece of toasted whole grain bread smeared with grass-fed butter.

CREAMY COCONUT RICE PUDDING

1½ cups cooked brown rice

1 cup coconut milk

½ cup almond or other milk

3 tablespoons shredded dried coconut

1/3 cup maple syrup

¼ cup raisins

1/8 teaspoon cinnamon

¼ cup chopped almonds, roasted

Preparation:

1. Combine all ingredients, except almonds, in a pot and cook over medium heat 7 to 10 minutes, or until creamy.
2. Garnish with roasted almonds.
3. Best served warm.

Menu Plan #5

	Main Meal	Leftovers	Leftovers
Breakfast	Soak black beans	Fried Polenta Squares	
Lunch		Seasonal Bean Salad in Lettuce Cups	Leftover Black Bean Soup with Whole Grain Bread
Dinner	Basic Black Beans Polenta With Sautéed Shitake Mushrooms and Turkey Sausage	Spicy Black Bean Soup with Polenta Croutons	Date night - go out with someone you love for a fabulous meal at your favorite restaurant

There are so many recipes and meals to choose from in each of these menus. The more you actively get into the kitchen and cook, the more proficient you can become, and the easier each cooking task will be. The best benefit of all ... better health can be yours with each delicious mouthful!

1. Make a big pot of Basic Black Beans plus Polenta with Sautéed Shitake Mushrooms and Turkey Sausage for dinner.
2. The next morning, you could fry up leftover polenta for a quick breakfast.

3. Make a light Seasonal Bean Salad in Lettuce Cups for lunch.
4. Prepare a Spicy Black Bean Soup with Polenta Croutons for dinner.
5. Freeze half of the soup to ensure you'll have food available the following week or at any other time during the month. The soup will stay good for 2 to 3 months in the freezer.
6. The next day, enjoy leftover Black Bean Soup and a honkin' hunk of whole grain bread smeared with grass-fed butter for lunch.
7. Date night! Whether you are married, engaged, or single, take yourself out for a fabulous meal at your favorite restaurant. You are worth it! I will teach you, in the "Lifestyle Strategies of the Healthy and Fabulous" chapter, how to make healthful and delicious choices when dining out.

BASIC BLACK BEANS

2 cups black turtle beans soaked in water to cover for 8 to 10 hours with a piece of kombu (sea vegetable)
4 cups water
2 bay leaves
1 teaspoon sea salt

Preparation:

1. Drain beans and discard soaking water (Do not discard kombu).
2. Put beans and water into a pot and bring to a boil.
3. Skim and discard foam that rises to the top.
4. Add bay leaves and reserved kombu to the pot.
5. Cover and reduce heat. Simmer 45 to 50 minutes.
6. Add sea salt and continue cooking 30 to 45 minutes or until beans soften.
7. Remove and discard bay leaves before serving.

POLENTA WITH SAUTÉED SHITAKE MUSHROOMS AND TURKEY SAUSAGE

3 cups water or chicken stock
1 cup cornmeal
1 teaspoon sea salt, divided
2 tablespoons butter or olive oil
1 large onion, peeled and diced or 3 to 4 spring onions or 1 leek, chopped)
10 to 12 shitake mushrooms (or any other type of mushroom), thinly sliced
½ pound ground turkey sausage
½ cup chicken or other stock
1/2 teaspoon dried tarragon
1 teaspoon dried thyme

Preparation:

1. In a medium pot, combine water and cornmeal. Bring to a boil.
2. Reduce heat to medium-low; add 1/2 teaspoon sea salt.
3. Cook, uncovered, 20 to 25 minutes, stirring to prevent lumps, until polenta is thick and bubbling.
4. Heat butter in a frying pan and sauté onion for 1 to 2 minutes.
5. Add mushrooms and continue cooking 2 to 3 minutes.
6. Add ground turkey sausage, breaking it into small pieces as it cooks.
7. Add chicken stock, remaining ½ teaspoon sea salt, tarragon, and thyme.
8. Put cooked polenta into a 9- x 13-inch casserole dish and let cool 10 to 15 minutes until firm to thc touch.
9. Cut polenta into squares, and top with sautéed vegetables and sausage.

FRIED POLENTA SQUARES

For those people craving corn muffins with a smear of butter in the morning, this is a great homemade alternative. It is basically the same ingredients (corn and butter) except… you're making it at home and adding in the flavor of LOVE!

1 to 2 tablespoons butter, schmaltz or other fat
Cooked polenta (can use cooked polenta from a natural foods market or grocery store)
Sea salt

Preparation:

1. Heat butter in a skillet.
2. Cut polenta into brownie-size squares.
3. If using store-bought polenta, cut into 1-inch thick round disks.
4. Season with salt and fry on medium heat 2 to 3 minutes on each side, or until lightly browned and crispy.

SEASONAL BEAN SALAD IN LETTUCE CUPS

1 cup fresh green beans, trimmed and cut into 2-inch pieces
2 yellow summer squash, cut into 1-inch rounds
1 small red onion, peeled and diced
8 to 10 cherry tomatoes, halved
1½ cups cooked black beans, or rinsed and drained canned beans
4 to 5 fresh basil leaves, thinly sliced
3 to 4 tablespoons extra virgin olive oil
2 tablespoons white wine vinegar or other vinegar
½ tablespoon local honey
1 teaspoon prepared mustard
Sea salt
Freshly ground black pepper
Butter Lettuce (or other lettuce)

Preparation:

1. Bring 2-inches water to boil in a pot with a steamer basket.
2. Add green beans. Cover and steam 2 to 3 minutes or until tender.
3. Remove green beans, drain, and set aside in a bowl.
4. Repeat steaming preparation with summer squash.
5. In a large bowl, combine green beans, summer squash, red onion, cherry tomatoes, black beans, and basil.
6. In a small bowl, whisk olive oil, vinegar, honey, mustard, and salt and pepper to taste.
7. Combine dressing with bean salad. Cover and marinate one hour or overnight in the refrigerator.
8. Separate lettuce leaves, rinse, and pat dry.
9. Spoon bean salad into the lettuce leaves (use the leaves as dainty little cups).

SPICY BLACK BEAN SOUP WITH POLENTA CROUTONS

1 tablespoon olive oil

1 onion, peeled and diced

2 garlic cloves, peeled and minced

1 teaspoon cumin

2 carrots, diced

1 celery stalk, diced

1 red bell pepper, seeded and diced

1 jalapeno pepper, seeded and diced

2 cups cooked black beans or rinsed and drained canned beans

4 cups chicken stock, beef stock, or water

Sea salt

3 to 4 tablespoons coconut oil

Cooked polenta (use leftover polenta or purchase pre-cooked polenta)

¼ cup chopped fresh cilantro

Preparation:

1. In a skillet, heat oil and sauté onion, garlic, and cumin 1 to 2 minutes.
2. Add carrots, celery, bell pepper, jalapeno, black beans and chicken stock.
3. Bring to a boil, add 1 teaspoon sea salt, cover, and simmer over medium-low heat for 5 to 7 minutes.
4. While bean soup is cooking, heat the coconut oil in a frying pan over medium heat.
5. Dice polenta into one-inch cubes and fry until lightly browned and crispy.
6. Drain polenta croutons on paper towels to remove excess oil.
7. Season the croutons with a pinch or two of sea salt.
8. Add cilantro to the soup at the end of cooking.
9. Ladle soup into bowls and top with polenta croutons.

Main Meal #6

	Main Meal	Leftovers	Leftovers
Breakfast		Savory Couscous Porridge	
Lunch	Marinate turkey in olive oil, herbs, and lemon juice	Prepare Turkey Stock (follow directions in stock chapter)	Creamy Turkey Chowder
Dinner	Whole Grain Couscous with Dried Cranberries Roasted Turkey with Herbed Gravy Sautéed Collard Greens with Garlic	Turkey and Kamut Pasta Salad with Homemade Mayonnaise	Hot Opened Turkey Sandwich On Whole Grain Bread, with Herbed Gravy

Turkey is usually eaten as holiday fare because it's a BIG bird that serves the masses of hungry relatives. But, turkey doesn't have to be eaten solely on the holidays. It can be enjoyed year round. To make preparation easier, purchase a whole turkey and have the butcher break it down for you. Or, if you are adept with a cleaver, break it down yourself. You can cook half a turkey or pieces of turkey instead of the entire bird to make the task less laborious.

1. Prepare Roasted Turkey with Herbed Gravy, Whole Grain Couscous with Dried Cranberries, and Sautéed Collard Greens with Garlic for dinner.
2. In the morning, prepare a quick-cooking Savory Couscous Porridge.
3. Bones and scraps from turkey can be used to make a nutritious pot of turkey stock.
4. Leftover turkey meat can be used to make a fun Turkey and Pasta Salad.
5. Turkey stock and turkey meat can be used to make Creamy Turkey Chowder.
6. Create Hot Opened Turkey Sandwiches with Herbed Gravy for dinner. It is the ultimate comfort food! Depending on the time of year, you could add a side salad (Spring, Summer) or roasted veggies (Fall, Winter).

WHOLE GRAIN COUSCOUS WITH DRIED CRANBERRIES

3 cups water or chicken stock

1 tablespoon butter

1 cup whole wheat couscous

¼ cup dried cranberries

¼ teaspoon sea salt

Preparation:

1. Bring water and butter to a boil in a medium saucepot.
2. Add couscous, dried cranberries, and salt.
3. Cook on high heat 2 to 3 minutes.
4. Remove from heat and let sit in the pot, covered, for 5 minutes.
5. Fluff with a fork and serve.

ROASTED TURKEY WITH HERBED GRAVY

2 to 3 tablespoons butter, softened
1 tablespoon each minced fresh rosemary, sage, and thyme,
Pastured or naturally raised whole turkey, ½ a turkey, or turkey pieces
Sea salt
Freshly ground black pepper
¼ cup cold water
2 to 3 tablespoons all purpose flour
1 tablespoon fresh herbs (your choice) or 1 teaspoon dried

Preparation:

1. Preheat oven to 375° F.
2. In a small bowl, combine butter and fresh herbs.
3. Smear herbed butter under the skin of the turkey.
4. Place turkey in roasting pan. Season with salt and pepper to taste. Cover tightly with aluminum foil.
5. Roast 15 to 18 minutes per pound of turkey.
6. Turn up the oven to 425 ° F, uncover, and continue roasting the turkey "open" during the last 45 minutes of cooking.
7. Baste the turkey with its own juices from the pan to brown and crisp the skin. If you do not enjoy eating skin, keep the turkey covered to ensure a moist finished product.
8. Let turkey rest in the pan for one-third the actual cooking time (e.g. if turkey took 1½ hours to cook, rest it for ½ an hour).
9. Transfer turkey to a large plate.
10. Pour turkey juices, fat, and herbs from the bottom of the roasting pan into a measuring cup.

11. Use 1 tablespoon flour per cup of liquid.
12. In a small bowl, combine cold water and flour, and add to the sauce pan along with the herbs.
13. Bring to a boil and cook 3 to 5 minutes or until gravy thickens.
14. If gravy is not thick enough, add more flour and water (remember to combine the flour with cold water before adding to the hot gravy otherwise it'll be lump-city).
15. Season to taste with salt and pepper.

SAVORY COUSCOUS PORRIDGE

¾ cup cooked couscous or 1/3 cup uncooked
1½ cups water or milk (whole milk, almond milk, etc.)
2 tablespoons butter
Pinch cinnamon
Pinch nutmeg
Pinch sea salt

Preparation:

1. In a medium pot, bring couscous, water, butter, cinnamon, nutmeg, and sea salt to a boil.
2. Lower heat to simmer and cook, covered, 5 to 7 minutes, or until creamy.

SAUTÉED COLLARD GREENS WITH GARLIC

1/3 cup water or stock
3 to 4 collard green leaves, thinly sliced
1 garlic clove, minced
2 teaspoons olive oil
Sea salt

Preparation:

1. Put water and collard greens into a frying pan over high heat and bring to a boil.
2. Cover, reduce heat, and steam 2 to 3 minutes, or until most of the liquid evaporates.
3. Add garlic, olive oil, and a pinch of salt.
4. Continue cooking 2 to 3 minutes, or until collards are bright green and tender.

TURKEY AND PASTA SALAD

1 cup whole grain elbow noodles (spelt, kamut, etc.)
1 teaspoon minced fresh sage
½ pound cooked naturally raised turkey, diced into bite-size pieces (about 1 cup)
2 to 3 celery stalks, finely diced
¼ cup dried cranberries
3 tablespoons Homemade Mayo (see following page), or store-bought mayonnaise
Sea salt
Freshly ground black pepper

Preparation:

1. In a large pot, cook noodles in boiling water according to package directions.
2. In a small bowl, mix sage into mayo until combined.
3. Drain pasta and put into a mixing bowl.
4. Combine pasta with turkey, celery, cranberries, and herbed mayo.
5. Season with salt and pepper to taste.

HOMEMADE MAYO

1 pastured or naturally grown egg, at room temperature, plus 1 egg yolk, at room temperature

1 teaspoon prepared mustard

1 tablespoon freshly squeezed lemon juice

1/4 teaspoon salt

3/4 cup olive oil

Preparation:

1. Eggs must be at room temperature.
2. Put eggs, mustard, lemon juice, and salt into a food processor and whip on high speed.
3. While the processor is on high, slowly add olive oil, a little bit at a time.
4. Continue until all the oil has been used and the mayo is thick and creamy.
5. Store in a jar, refrigerated, 7 to 10 days.

CREAMY TURKEY CHOWDER

2 to 3 tablespoons grass-fed butter
2 to 3 tablespoons white rice flour (or other flour)
4 cups turkey or chicken stock
1 leek, chopped (use both white and green parts)
1 tablespoon minced fresh sage
1 teaspoon dried rosemary
2 to 3 garlic cloves, peeled and minced
½ cup celeriac root, peeled diced (or 2 celery stalks, diced)
2 carrots, diced
1 large Yukon gold potato, diced
1 teaspoon sea salt
Freshly ground black pepper
1½ cup cooked turkey pieces, diced
1 tablespoon minced fresh parsley

Preparation:

1. In a medium pot, heat butter and flour together.
2. Add stock and whisk until combined.
3. Add leek, sage, rosemary, garlic, celeriac root, carrots, potato, salt, and pepper to taste.
4. Cover and bring to a boil.
5. Reduce heat to medium and cook 15 to 18 minutes.
6. Add diced turkey and parsley.
7. Cook an additional 1 to 2 minutes. Adjust seasoning to taste.

HOT OPENED TURKEY SANDWICHES WITH HERBED GRAVY

Whole Grain Bread (1 to 2 slices per person)

Boneless turkey meat

Herbed Gravy

Preparation:

1. Lay bread flat on a plate.
2. Warm the turkey pieces in the oven or on the stove top.
3. Place warm turkey on top of bread.
4. Cover with spoonfuls of hot Herbed Gravy.

HERBED GRAVY

½ teaspoon dried thyme

¼ teaspoon dried sage

1/4 teaspoon dried rosemary

2 tablespoons butter

1 cup chicken or turkey stock

1 to 2 tablespoons all purpose flour

¼ cup cold water

Sea salt

Freshly ground black pepper

Preparation:

1. In a frying pan or small saucepot, sauté herbs 2 to 3 minutes in butter.
2. Add stock.
3. In a small bowl, combine all purpose flour with cold water and add to the pot.
4. Season with salt and pepper to taste.
5. Cook over medium-high heat until gravy thickens.

Menu Plan #7

	Main Meal	Leftovers	Leftovers
Breakfast	Break down duck into pieces (legs, wings, breasts, etc.) and prepare duck stock		
Lunch	Render duck fat from excess skin and fat	Savory Shitake Mushroom Soup	Duck Liver Pâté on Whole Grain Toast
Dinner	Braised Duck with Tahini Noodles Hearty Roasted Winter Roots Sautéed Brussels Sprouts with Cranberries and Almonds	Pan-Seared Duck Breast & Chinese Cabbage Salad with Crunchy Cracklins	Caramelized Onion Soup

Duck is one of my all-time favorite foods in the fall and winter. It is a hearty, warming food and is rich in good fat. Like all poultry, duck fat is mainly monounsaturated fat and is low in polyunsaturated fat, which makes it a good fat for frying. Some people are afraid of eating duck because of its high fat content -- but fear not. Let's follow the lead of the French and Chinese who have enjoyed duck for centuries and have also enjoyed long healthy lives.

1. Purchase one whole duck and break it down into pieces (legs, thighs, wings, breasts, and carcass); or have the butcher break it down for you.
2. Make duck stock using carcass and neck.
3. Remove some of the skin and fat from the duck to render fat for cooking.
4. For dinner, prepare Tahini Noodles & Braised Duck, Hearty Roasted Winter Roots, and Sautéed Brussels Sprouts with Cranberry and Almonds.
5. The following day prepare Savory Shitake Mushroom Soup with the delicious duck stock.
6. Prepare Pan-Seared Duck Breast & Chinese Cabbage Salad with Crunchy Cracklins.
7. Use duck liver for a small amount of pâté, or freeze livers until you have acquired enough to make a larger portion (2 to 3 duck livers).
8. Make a yummy Caramelized Onion Soup with duck stock!

TAHINI NOODLES & BRAISED DUCK

2 each duck legs, thighs, and wings, skin removed

2 to 3 cups chicken stock or water

2 inches ginger, thinly sliced

1½ tablespoons tamari (or naturally fermented soy sauce)

1 (8.8 ounces) package udon noodles

3 tablespoons tahini

2 tablespoons shoyu

2 tablespoons brown rice vinegar

1½ tablespoons maple syrup

1 garlic clove, peeled and chopped

Dash cayenne pepper

½ cup water

2 scallions, minced

1 sheet nori sea vegetable, toasted and crumbled

Preparation:

1. Place duck pieces, stock, ginger, and tamari in a large pot. Make sure duck is covered with liquid. Bring to boil.
2. Reduce heat to medium-low.
3. Cover and cook one hour, turning the pieces one time midway through cooking.
4. Continue cooking until most of the liquid evaporates.
5. Let duck cool and shred meat with a fork.
6. Cook noodles according to instructions on package.
7. In a food processor combine tahini, shoyu, brown rice vinegar, maple syrup, garlic, cayenne pepper, and water.
8. Combine tahini dressing with noodles, shredded duck, and minced scallions.
9. Garnish with toasted nori.

RENDERED DUCK FAT

Duck fat is a great fat for frying and baking because it is stable at high temperatures. It's also considered a healthful fat. "All poultry fats contain the monounsaturated fatty acid palmitoleic acid, which is believed to boost our immune system."[37] I render duck fat every time I purchase a duck. The fat keeps in the refrigerator for up to two months, or in the freezer for up to six months.

Duck fat, skin, and tail

Preparation:

1. Trim excess skin and fat from duck, and chop into small pieces.
2. Chop tail into smaller pieces.
3. Heat a skillet or frying pan over low heat.
4. Place duck skin, fat, and tail into the pan and cook slowly until fat becomes liquid.
5. Strain fat using a cheese cloth or fine mesh strainer.
6. Reserve fat in a glass jar or other container.
7. Duck fat and other poultry fats can keep in the refrigerator for up to two months.
8. You can also render the fat from chicken using this same method – Chicken fat is called schmaltz.

---

[37] FAT, An Appreciation of a Misunderstood Ingredient, Jennifer McLagan, Ten Speed Press, 2008, p. 123

PAN-SEARED DUCK BREAST & CHINESE CABBAGE SALAD WITH CRUNCHY CRACKLINS

2 duck breasts
Sea salt
Freshly ground black pepper
1 head Chinese cabbage, shredded
2 carrots, grated or cut into thin matchsticks
2 to 3 scallions, minced
6 tablespoons toasted sesame oil
4 tablespoons brown rice vinegar (or other vinegar)
1 tablespoon ginger juice (grate fresh ginger and squeeze out juice)

Preparation:

1. Remove fatty skin from duck breast and chop into ½-inch pieces.
2. Heat a frying pan on very low heat and add fatty duck skin.
3. Fat will render from the duck skin.
4. Continue cooking pieces of skin in the fat until lightly browned.
5. Remove cracklins (duck skin pieces) from the frying pan and drain on a paper towel.
6. Season cracklins with a pinch of sea salt while still hot.
7. Season duck breast with salt and pepper to taste and place on top of the rendered duck fat in the hot pan.
8. Cook over medium heat for 3 to 4 minutes on each side.
9. Transfer duck onto a plate and let it rest for 5 to 7 minutes.
10. While duck breast is resting, combine Chinese cabbage, carrots, and scallions in a large bowl.

11. In a small bowl, whisk toasted sesame oil, brown rice vinegar, ginger juice, and a couple of pinches of sea salt.
12. Cut duck breast into ¼-inch slices and add to the salad.
13. Toss salad with dressing.
14. Garnish salad with crispy cracklins.

HEARTY ROASTED WINTER ROOTS

3 carrots, chopped into thick chunks

2 parsnips, chopped into thick chunks

2 turnips, diced

2 tablespoons schmaltz, duck fat, or olive oil

Sea salt

Freshly ground black pepper

1 tablespoon minced fresh parsley

Preparation:

1. Preheat oven to 400° F.
2. Combine carrots, parsnips, and turnips in a casserole dish and coat evenly with duck fat.
3. Season with salt and pepper to taste.
4. Cover tightly and roast 30 minutes.
5. Uncover and roast an additional 20 to 25 minutes.
6. Garnish with parsley.

SAUTÉED BRUSSELS SPROUTS WITH CRANBERRIES & TOASTED ALMONDS

1/3 cup water or stock

1 pint Brussels sprouts (10 to 12), cleaned and halved

¼ cup dried cranberries

Sea salt

1 tablespoon olive oil

¼ cup chopped almonds, toasted

Preparation:

1. In a frying pan, bring water, Brussels sprouts, and cranberries to a boil. Add a couple of pinches of sea salt.
2. Cover and cook 5 to 7 minutes or until liquid evaporates.
3. Drizzle with olive oil and toss with toasted almonds.
4. Continue cooking 3 to 5 minutes to caramelize Brussels sprouts.

SAVORY SHITAKE MUSHROOM SOUP

1 large onion, peeled and diced
1 tablespoon butter
1 teaspoon dried tarragon
8 ounces fresh cremini mushrooms, chopped (approximately 4 cups)
8 ounces fresh shitake mushrooms, chopped (approximately 2 cups)
4 cups duck or chicken stock
1 teaspoon sea salt
Fresh chives, minced

Preparation:

1. Sauté onion in butter in a frying pan for 2 to 3 minutes.
2. Add tarragon, mushrooms, stock, and sea salt, and bring to a boil.
3. Cover and cook on medium heat 7 to 10 minutes.
4. Remove onions and mushrooms from soup with a slotted spoon and puree in a food processor or blender until smooth.
5. Return puree to the broth.
6. Place into individual dishes and garnish with fresh chives.

DUCK LIVER PÂTÉ

2 shallots, peeled and minced
1 garlic clove, peeled and minced
1 teaspoon fresh thyme or ½ teaspoon dried
3 tablespoons rendered duck fat or butter
2 to 3 duck livers
1 tablespoon brandy or 2 tablespoons white wine
Sea salt
4 tablespoons butter, softened
Whole grain toast or whole grain crackers

Preparation:

1. In a skillet, sauté shallots, garlic, and thyme in fat for 2 to 3 minutes.
2. Add duck livers, brandy, and a generous pinch of sea salt.
3. Cook livers 2 minutes on each side.
4. Put all ingredients plus butter into the food processor and puree until smooth and creamy.
5. Transfer into a small container and let set at least 1½ to 2 hours in the refrigerator.
6. Enjoy a healthy shmear or two on your favorite crackers or whole grain bread.

CARAMELIZED ONION SOUP

This is my version of French onion soup. Omigosh, it's totally yummy! Taste it and let me know your thoughts. You can email me at my website (www.AndreaBeaman.com) with comments or questions about this or any other recipe in this book.

3 large onions (Vidalia, yellow, white, or red), peeled and diced
1 tablespoon duck or chicken fat, olive oil, or butter
2 garlic cloves, peeled and minced
½ cup Mirin rice cooking wine (or any white wine)
4 cups duck stock
1 teaspoon fresh thyme or ½ teaspoon dried
2 bay leaves
1 teaspoon sea salt

Preparation:

1. In a skillet over low heat, sauté onions in duck fat for 15 minutes.
2. Stir the onions a few times to ensure they do not burn.
3. Add garlic and mirin, and continue cooking 10 to 15 minutes until onions caramelize and turn light brown. Do not let them burn.
4. Add stock, thyme, bay leaves, and sea salt, and bring to a boil.
5. Cover and cook over medium-low heat for 15 minutes.
6. Adjust seasonings if needed. Remove and discard bay leaves before serving.

Chapter 10

THE POT OF GOLD

The pot of gold at the end of the rainbow doesn't have to be an elusive fantasy. It can be a reality. We need only to slightly alter our perception of what is actually *inside* that pot. Use your imagination here: Picture a piping hot pot of scrumptious slowly simmered food that magically fuels your body with yummy homemade goodness. Now, that's what I call a pot of gold!

Wonderful one-pot meals make it possible to enjoy fully balanced dinners (lunches and breakfasts too) without all the muss and fuss and dirty dishes. How many of us can honestly say we enjoy washing pots and pans? Probably not too many. As a matter of fact, one of the biggest complaints from clients (besides lacking time to get into the kitchen and cook!) is that they hate dealing with the cleanup. Ugh! Nothing elicits heartburn quicker than staring at a sink full of dishes piled ten feet high.

The one-pot meals in this chapter are all, simply, cooked in ONE POT. Not kidding, totally serious, I'm not pulling your leg here. One-pot means one pot! Put the antacids away; there will be no heartburn tonight. I know you can handle the task of cleaning one paltry pot.

Some people may not understand the concept of One-Pot Meals, so I'm here to cut through the confusion. On a popular television show, *Top Chef* (Season 5, episode 6), Martha Stewart judged the cheftestants on their ability to prepare a one-pot meal in under one hour.

Many of the chefs used one pot to create one element of the dish, and then cleaned it out and used it over and over again to create each additional element. They used their one pot three and four times. Yikes! I was flabbergasted when Martha Stewart chose the herb-rubbed filet mignon with cauliflower puree as the winning dish. Although I'm sure it was delectable, it was *not* a one-pot meal. In addition to cleaning and reusing the pot repeatedly, the chef added a food processor into the mix to puree the cauliflower. This is clearly not a one-pot meal. The dish that probably should have won the challenge was the one-pot paella. The chef simply used one pot, one time, to make one delicious dish. Martha, Martha, Martha! What the heck were you thinking? We may need to send you back to the "big house" for that culinary scandal.

This chapter demonstrates how to make fully balanced meals that are truly cooked in one pot. Nice, easy, breezy cooking. Many of my clients work full-time jobs (outside the home) and the thought of preparing food after a long day at the office simply paralyzes them. The only part of their bodies functioning during this traumatic time is one finger used to dial Chinese food delivery.

It's at times like this that a slow cooker comes to the rescue. It lets you prepare meals without having to babysit the food. Simply place the ingredients into a slow cooker before leaving for work in the morning. Set the timer on low for 10 hours. By the time you return home, all you need to do is lift the lid, ladle your home-cooked goodies into a bowl, and serve. Voila! If you feel the need, you could pair your one-pot meal with a side salad or slice of whole grain bread; but mostly, it is a balanced meal exactly as it is.

The recipes in this section can be prepared in a large soup pot or in a slow cooker. I will give directions for both cooking options where appropriate.

Don't wait for that elusive little leprechaun to magically appear and tell you where the pot of gold is; get your apron on, and cook your way to the end of the rainbow!

MAGNIFICENT MINESTRONG!

No, that's not a typo. This soup is called "Minestrong." With the addition of traditional beef stock as the base, you'll receive a host of beneficial bone-building nutrients. Yeah baby, strengthen your bones with every bowlful!

1 tablespoon butter
1 tablespoon olive oil
1 leek, cleaned and chopped (use white and green parts)
3 to 4 garlic cloves, peeled and diced
2 carrots, sliced into ¼-inch rounds
1 celery stalk, diced
½ cup canned diced tomatoes, undrained
5 cups beef bone stock (can substitute chicken, turkey, etc.)
1½ teaspoons sea salt
1 teaspoon dried thyme leaves
½ teaspoon dried rosemary
½ cup kamut elbow pasta or other pasta
1½ cups cooked kidney beans or one (15-ounce) can, rinsed and drained
2 leaves Swiss chard, chopped
Parmigiano Reggiano (optional)

Preparation:

1. In a soup pot, heat butter and oil and sauté leeks for 2 to 3 minutes.
2. Add garlic, carrots, celery, tomatoes, stock, salt, thyme, and rosemary.
3. Cover and cook over medium-high heat for 5 to 7 minutes.
4. Add pasta, beans, and Swiss chard.
5. Bring soup back up to a boil.
6. Reduce heat to low for an additional 10 to 12 minutes.
7. Garnish with shaved Parmigiano Reggiano.

Slow Cooker Preparation:

1. Put all ingredients except pasta and Parmigiano Reggiano into a slow cooker, using 4 cups of stock instead 5.
2. Cook on low-heat setting for 8 hours, or on high-heat setting for 3 to 4 hours.
3. Add pasta during the last 20 minutes of cooking.
4. Garnish with freshly grated Parmigiano Reggiano.

HEARTY LENTIL STEW

2 tablespoons olive oil or 1 tablespoon chicken fat

1 leek, cleaned and cut into 1-inch pieces (use both white and green part)

2 garlic cloves, peeled and minced

5 cups chicken stock or water

3 cups cooked lentils, or 2 (15-ounce) cans, rinsed and drained

2 parsnips, in ½-inch dice

3 carrots, in ½-inch dice

1 medium celeriac root, peeled, and chopped in ½-inch dice

1 Yukon gold potato, in ½-inch dice

2 tablespoons minced fresh thyme leaves

1½ teaspoons sea salt

¼ teaspoon freshly ground black pepper

2 links cooked pork or turkey sausage (4 links), diced

1/4 cup minced parsley

Preparation:

1. In a large pot, heat oil, and sauté leeks and garlic 2 to 3 minutes.
2. Add chicken stock, lentils, parsnips, carrots, celeriac root, potatoes, thyme, salt, and pepper.
3. Cover and bring to a boil.
4. Reduce heat to medium, and cook 20 to 25 minutes.
5. Remove one-third of the ingredients and puree in a food processor or blender.
6. Return the puree to the soup.
7. Add sausage and parsley, and cook an additional 3 to 4 minutes.

Slow Cooker Preparation:

1. Put all ingredients except parsley into a slow cooker, using 4 cups of stock instead 5.
2. Cook on high heat 4 hours, or low heat for 8 hours.
3. Garnish with parsley before serving.

SAVORY TURKEY CHILI

1 tablespoon olive oil or chicken fat (schmaltz)

1 onion, peeled and diced

2 garlic cloves, peeled and minced

1/2 pound ground pastured, naturally raised turkey meat

1 red pepper, seeded and diced

1 poblano pepper, seeded and diced

2 tomatoes, chopped into chunks

2 teaspoons fresh thyme leaves

1 tablespoon fresh savory leaves

½ teaspoon sea salt

3 cups cooked pinto beans, or 2 (15-ounce) cans, rinsed and drained

1 cup turkey stock or other stock

Raw milk cheddar cheese, grated

Preparation:

1. In a large frying pan or pot, heat oil and sauté onions and garlic for 2 to 3 minutes.
2. Add ground turkey, breaking it up into small pieces as it cooks, 3 to 4 minutes.
3. Add red pepper, poblano pepper, tomatoes, thyme, savory, sea salt, beans, and turkey stock.
4. Cover, and cook over medium heat for 1/2 hour.
5. Garnish individual bowls with grated cheddar cheese.

Slow Cooker Preparation:

1. Put onions, garlic, oil, peppers, tomatoes, thyme, savory, salt, and beans into a slow cooker.
2. Pull ground turkey apart with your fingers and add to the slow cooker in small pieces.
3. Add turkey stock.
4. Cover and cook on high heat 4 hours, or low heat 7 to 8 hours.
5. Garnish with grated cheddar cheese.

ONE-POT WILD SALMON STEW

5 cups water or fish stock
1 inch ginger, peeled and cut into matchsticks
1 red onion, peeled and cut into large chunks
2 carrots, thickly cut on the diagonal
½ cup butternut or buttercup squash, diced
4 to 5 shitake mushrooms, thinly sliced
1 stalk broccoli florets and stem, (slice stem into thin rounds)
6 to 7 ounces wild salmon (or other fish), cut into 2-ounce pieces
2 to 3 kale leaves, cut into bite-size pieces
4 tablespoons white miso or chick pea miso
2 cups leftover grains (brown rice, noodles, etc.)
¼ bunch watercress

Preparation:

1. In a large pot, bring water, ginger, onions, carrots, squash, and mushrooms to a boil.
2. Reduce heat, cover, and cook over medium heat 5 to 7 minutes.
3. Add broccoli and cook 1 to 2 minutes.
4. Add salmon and cook 2 to 3 minutes.
5. Add kale and cook 2 to 3 minutes, or until bright green.
6. Dilute miso in a small amount of water and add to the soup.
7. Add grains and continue cooking 2 to 3 minutes.
8. Ladle into large bowls and garnish with fresh watercress.

Slow Cooker Preparation:

1. Put water, ginger, onions, carrots, squash, mushrooms, broccoli, and kale into the slow cooker.
2. Cook on high temperature 4 hours, or low 6 to 7 hours.
3. During the last 20 minutes of cooking, add salmon.
4. In a small bowl, dilute miso in a small amount of water and add to slow cooker.
5. Add grains to the slow cooker and continue cooking until all ingredients are cooked.
6. Garnish with fresh watercress.

SEA BASS SOUP WITH SOBA NOODLES

5 cups water or fish stock
1 leek, cleaned and cut thickly on the diagonal (use both white and green parts)
2 inches ginger, peeled and cut into thin matchsticks
1 cup roughly chopped green cabbage
1 carrot, cut into ¼-inch diagonals
12 to 16 ounces black sea bass or black cod, with skin, cut into 4 equal pieces
½ (8-ounce) package soba noodles
4 tablespoons sweet white miso
3 to 4 bok choy leaves, chopped into bite-size pieces
1 sheet toasted nori seaweed, cut into thin slivers

Preparation:

1. In a large pot, bring water, leeks, ginger, cabbage, and carrots to a boil.
2. Reduce heat to low, and cook 5 to 7 minutes.
3. Add fish and noodles, cover, and cook 3 minutes.
4. In a small bowl, dilute the miso paste with water or broth from soup.
5. Add bok choy and diluted miso to soup, cover, and cook 3 to 4 minutes over low heat.
6. Ladle soup, noodles, and a piece of fish into individual bowls.
7. Garnish with a few slivers of nori sea vegetable.

WINTER WHITE BEAN STEW

2 cups cooked cannellini beans or 1 (15-ounce) can, rinsed and drained

4 cups chicken stock

2 bay leaves

1½ teaspoons sea salt

1 onion, peeled and diced

2 carrots, diced

½ celery root (celeriac), peeled and diced

3 roasted or fresh garlic cloves

½ teaspoon dried rosemary

1 teaspoon dried thyme leaves

Freshly ground black pepper

½ cup whole grain or semolina pasta

2 to 3 kale leaves, ripped into bite-size pieces

1 to 2 tablespoons minced fresh parsley

Preparation:

1. In a large pot, bring to a boil beans, stock, bay leaves, salt, onions, carrots, celery root, garlic, rosemary, thyme, and pepper to taste.
2. Cover, reduce heat, and cook 20 to 25 minutes.
3. Add pasta and kale, and cook an additional 7 to 10 minutes.
4. Remove and discard bay leaves.
5. Ladle into serving bowls and garnish with parsley.

Slow Cooker Preparation:

1. Put all ingredients except kale and pasta into a slow cooker.
2. Cook on low-heat setting for 8 hours, or on high-heat setting for 4 hours.
3. Add kale and pasta during the last 20 minutes of cooking.
4. Garnish with parsley.

CHUNKY CHICKEN SOUP

5 cups chicken stock or water
1 onion, peeled and diced
1 small celeriac root, peeled and diced
3 carrots, diced
1 medium Yukon gold or red potato, diced
Organic, pastured chicken pieces with bones (wings, drumsticks, carcass, etc.)
1 tablespoon fresh thyme leaves
1½ teaspoons sea salt
2 tablespoons minced fresh parsley
2 to 3 garlic cloves, peeled and minced
½ cup alphabet pasta or other noodles

Preparation:

1. Bring stock, onions, celeraic root, carrots, potatoes, chicken, thyme, and sea salt to a boil in a large pot.
2. Reduce heat, cover, and simmer 35 to 40 minutes.
3. Add parsley, garlic, and pasta; continue cooking 7 to 10 minutes.

Slow Cooker Preparation:

1. Put 4 cups (instead of 5) stock, onions, celeraic root, carrots, potatoes, chicken, thyme, salt, and garlic into a slow cooker.
2. Cook on high heat 4 hours, or low heat 8 hours.
3. Add parsley and pasta during the last 20 minutes of cooking.

SUMMER VEGETABLES AND BEAN STEW

1 tablespoon olive oil
1 onion, peeled and diced
3 garlic cloves, peeled and minced
4 cups chicken stock
1 green zucchini, cut into ½-inch rounds
1 yellow summer squash, cut into ½-inch rounds
1 (15-ounce) can roasted tomatoes, undrained
1½ cups cooked cannelini beans, or 1 (15-ounce) can, rinsed and drained
1 teaspoon fresh oregano
1 teaspoon sea salt
1 tablespoon minced fresh basil
Shaved Parmigiano Reggiano

Preparation:

1. In a large pot, heat oil and sauté onions and garlic for 3 to 4 minutes.
2. Add stock, zucchini, summer squash, tomatoes, beans, oregano, and sea salt, and bring to a boil.
3. Cover and simmer 30 to 35 minutes.
4. Add basil, and cook an additional 2 to 3 minutes.
5. Garnish with shaved Parmigiano Reggiano.

Slow Cooker Preparation:

1. Put all ingredients except basil and Parmigiano Reggiano and basil, using 3 cups of stock instead 4, into a slow cooker.
2. Cook on low temperature 7 to 8 hours, or high temperature 3½ to 4 hours.
3. During the last 10 minutes of cooking, add basil.
4. Garnish individual bowls with Parmigiano Reggiano.

TEX-MEX CHILI CON CARNE

2 tablespoons olive oil
½ teaspoon ground coriander
½ teaspoon allspice
1 teaspoon cumin
2 garlic cloves, peeled and minced
1 large onion, peeled and diced
8 to 10 ounces sirloin steak, diced (can substitute ground beef)
1 jalapeño pepper, seeded and diced
2 tomatoes, seeded and diced
Kernels from 1 ear corn
1½ cups canned kidney beans, rinsed and drained
1½ cups canned black-eyed peas, rinsed and drained
½ cup water or stock (chicken, beef, or veggie)
1 teaspoon sea salt
Shredded Cheddar cheese
Minced chives

Preparation:

1. In a deep frying pan, heat oil and sauté coriander, allspice, and cumin for 1 minute.
2. Add garlic and onions, and sauté 2 to 3 minutes.
3. Add diced beef, and cook 1 minute, or until lightly browned.
4. Add jalapeño, tomatoes, corn, kidney beans, black-eyed peas, water, and sea salt.
5. Cover and bring to a boil.
6. Reduce heat to medium, and cook 25 to 35 minutes.
7. Garnish with cheddar cheese and minced chives.

Slow Cooker Preparation:

1. Put all ingredients except cheddar cheese and chives into the slow cooker.
2. Cook on high temperature 4 hours, or low 8 to 9 hours.
3. Garnish individual servings with cheddar cheese and chives.

BUFFALO CHILI

2 tablespoons olive oil, duck fat, or bacon fat
1 onion, peeled and diced
½ pound ground buffalo meat
1½ teaspoons cumin
1 teaspoon sea salt
¼ teaspoon freshly ground black pepper
3 celery stalks, diced
2 garlic cloves, peeled and minced
1 red pepper, seeded and diced
1½ cups cooked pinto beans, or 1 (15-ounce) can, rinsed and drained
1 (15-ounce) can crushed tomatoes, with liquid
½ cup water or beef stock
2 ounces blue cheese, crumbled

Preparation:

1. In a large pot, over medium heat, heat oil and sauté onions 2 to 3 minutes.
2. Add buffalo in small pieces to the pan and cook 1 to 2 minutes, breaking up meat as it cooks.
3. Add cumin, salt, pepper, celery, garlic, red pepper, beans, tomatoes, and water.
4. Bring to a boil. Cover, reduce heat to low, and simmer for 25 to 30 minutes.
5. Garnish with crumbled blue cheese.

Slow Cooker Preparation:

1. Put onions, oil, cumin, black pepper, celery, garlic, red pepper, pinto beans, tomatoes, and salt into a slow cooker.
2. Pull apart small pieces of ground buffalo meat and add to the pot.
3. Add 1 cup water or stock to the slow cooker.
4. Cover and cook on high temperature 4 hours, or on low temperature 8 to 9 hours.
5. Garnish individual bowls of chili with crumbled blue cheese.

HEARTY BEEF STEW

3 tablespoons whole grain flour
Sea salt
Freshly ground black pepper
Cayenne pepper
8 to 10 ounces grass-fed beef stew meat, cut into 1-inch chunks
1 tablespoon olive oil, duck fat, or chicken fat
1 onion, peeled and cut into thick wedges
4 carrots, cut into ½-inch pieces
3 small red potatoes, quartered
2 celery stalks, in ½-inch dice
3 to 4 button mushrooms, quartered
1 cup fresh stringbeans, cut into 2-inch pieces
3 cups beef or chicken stock
½ cup red wine
½ teaspoon dried thyme leaves

Preparation:

1. Put flour into a large plastic baggie.
2. Season with a couple of pinches of sea salt, black pepper, and cayenne pepper.
3. Drop the beef chunks into the baggie and coat evenly with flour.
4. In a soup pot, heat oil and sauté beef 1 minute on each side or until lightly browned.
5. Add onions, carrots, potatoes, celery, mushrooms, stringbeans, stock, wine, thyme, and ½ teaspoon salt.
6. Bring to a boil.
7. Reduce heat to medium-low, cover, and cook 45 to 50 minutes.

Slow Cooker Preparation:

1. Put all ingredients except seasoned flour into slow cooker, using 1 1/2 cups of stock instead 3.
2. Cover and cook on low temperature for 9 hours, or high temperature for 4½ hours.
3. One-half hour before cooking finishes, combine seasoned flour with a small amount of water (2 to 3 tablespoons) and add to the liquid in the slow cooker.
4. Cover and finish cooking until liquid thickens.

STEWED LAMB WITH APRICOTS

8 to 10 ounces pastured lamb stew meat, cubed
1 tablespoon olive oil, chicken fat, or duck fat
½ teaspoon cumin
½ teaspoon cinnamon
Dash ground nutmeg
1 tablespoon butter
6 to 8 dried apricots, diced
¼ cup raisins
2 onions, peeled and quartered
3 garlic cloves, peeled and chopped
½ teaspoon sea salt
1/8 teaspoon freshly ground black pepper
1½ cups water or stock
1½ cups red wine
1 sprig fresh parsley, chopped

Preparation:

1. In a large pot, sear lamb in fat until lightly browned on all sides.
2. Add cumin, cinnamon, nutmeg, butter, apricots, raisins, onions, garlic, salt, pepper, water, and wine to the pot.
3. Bring to a boil.
4. Cover, reduce heat to medium, and cook 45 to 50 minutes.
5. Add parsley at the end of cooking.

Slow Cooker Preparation:

1. Place ingredients into a slow cooker starting with butter at the bottom, onions, garlic, apricots, raisins, cumin, cinnamon, nutmeg, salt, pepper, 1 cup stock, wine, and the stew meat on top.
2. Cook in slow cooker on high temperature setting 4 to 5 hours, or on low temperature setting 8 to 10 hours.
3. Garnish with parsley.

Chapter 11

FROZEN ASSETS

It's not uncommon for people to eat directly out of their freezer. I know I did. When I was growing up in the 1970s and 1980s (omigosh... did I just date myself?), both mom and dad worked two jobs to support the family. We had a roof over our heads, clothes on our back, shoes on our feet, and lots of fun stuff to play with. There was only one thing missing: wholesome home-cooked food. While our parents worked long hours, we subsisted on frozen Hungry Man dinners, Swanson Chicken Pot Pies, Ellio's frozen pizzas, and other frosty fare. It was all highly processed, packaged, and stored in the electric mini-glacier until we were ready to heat it and eat it. These foods were quick and convenient, but most lacked good quality ingredients and were usually over salted.

Interestingly, the tastiest frozen foods were always the ones prepared and stored in the freezer by either mom or dad. Every few months, my dad made a gigantic vat of split pea soup with ham bone, and then froze half of it in large containers for future meals. Very smart! It cut down kitchen time and ensured there would be food available at a later date. Thanks for the wise tip, Daddy-O!

Anytime I make a pot of soup or stock, I freeze half of it (just like dad did) to use at a later date. It's comforting to know there is always something highly nutritious and ready to thaw, heat, and eat when needed. Any of the soups or stocks in previous chapters can be stored in the freezer. When storing, keep in mind that liquids expand. Leave about two inches of empty space before sealing and freezing liquids.

My freezer is also used for storing stock bones and animal proteins (meat, fish, chicken, sausages, etc.). Foods can keep safely in moisture-proof bags or freezer-safe containers (glass or plastic) for many months. Frozen foods can easily be neglected – out of sight, out of mind. It's a good idea to date and label any food before storing in the freezer. Otherwise you may find yourself digging out mysterious items that resemble a woolly mammoth or other creature from the ice age. A good rule of thumb: if you don't know what it is or how long it's been there, don't eat it. The freezer doesn't completely stop the breakdown process of food, it just slows it down. That means food can and does go bad inside the freezer.

You can safely freeze:

- Broths, soups, and stews for 2 to 3 months
- Freshly frozen meats and fish for 3 to 6 months
- After 6 months… we can certainly still eat the foods that have been frozen, but why on earth would we want to? If it's been in the freezer that long, it must not have tasted too good in the first place!

There are great quality packaged foods that can be *purchased* already frozen. For example, organic frozen mixed vegetables are good for quick and easy stir-fries and soups. Other frozen foods include spinach, asparagus, green beans, corn, broccoli, Asian vegetables, carrots, berries, and other fruits. I will show you what to do with these foods in the pages that follow.

Other quick and easy foods that can either be made and frozen or store-bought frozen include buffalo, turkey, beef, and salmon burgers; and bags of shrimp and fish, and packages of sausage links (chicken, turkey and pork).

I highly encourage you to prepare *fresh food* from local and seasonal products in order to make the best possible investment in your health. Fresh food is the ideal. If you don't have the time or access to that type of food, count on these frozen assets to help you out in the kitchen. If you are strapped for time and in a bind, reach into your freezer, excavate something (anything!), thaw it, and cook it. Any frozen food recipe in this chapter can be made with fresh food, too. I'll give examples of how to cook with both frozen and fresh.

Lastly, simply adding something fresh (not previously frozen), like a sprig of parsley or minced herbs, can help liven up a dish and give it a little life. Put your mittens on and let's get cooking!

CREAMY ASPARAGUS SOUP

1 (8- to 10-ounce) bag or box frozen organic asparagus or 1 bunch fresh asparagus (remove about 1 to 2 inches of the stem)
2 to 3 garlic cloves, peeled and diced
2 red potatoes, diced
1 leek, cleaned and chopped (white and green parts)
4 to 5 cups chicken, beef, veggie stock or water
1 teaspoon sea salt
½ red bell pepper, seeded and finely diced

Preparation:

1. Put asparagus, garlic, potatoes, leeks, stock, and salt into a large pot and bring to a boil.
2. Cover, reduce heat to medium, and cook 10 to 15 minutes, or until potato is tender.
3. Remove vegetables with a slotted spoon and puree in a food processor or blender.
4. Return vegetable back to the soup.
5. Serve in individual bowls garnished with red pepper.

SPRING PEA SOUP

1 tablespoon olive oil

2 large spring onions, white and green parts, diced, or 1 large onion, peeled and diced

1 (16-ounce) bag frozen green peas or 2 cups fresh green (English) peas

½ teaspoon dried rosemary

4 cups vegetable stock or water

1 teaspoon sea salt

Freshly ground black pepper

1 or 2 mint leaves, minced

Preparation:

- In a large pot, heat oil and sauté onions 1 to 2 minutes.
- Add green peas, rosemary, stock, and salt. Bring to a boil.
- Reduce heat to medium-low, cover, and cook 10 to 15 minutes
- Remove vegetables and puree in a food processor or blender.
- Return pureed vegetables back to the soup.
- Add freshly ground black pepper and adjust seasoning to taste.
- Garnish with mint.

SILKY CORN CHOWDER

2 tablespoons grass-fed butter
1 large onion, peeled and chopped
4 to 5 cups chicken or vegetable stock, or water
2 (16-ounce) bags frozen corn kernels or kernels from 4 ears fresh corn
1 teaspoon sea salt
1 tablespoon minced fresh cilantro

Preparation:

1. In a large pot, heat butter, and sauté onions 2 to 3 minutes.
2. Add stock and corn (If using fresh corn, put the kernels *and* the cobs into the water to infuse more corn flavor).
3. Cover and cook 7 to 10 minutes or until tender.
4. Remove and discard corn cobs.
5. Puree corn and onions in a food processor or blender.
6. Add pureed vegetables back to soup; add salt.
7. Cook 5 minutes on medium heat.
8. Garnish with cilantro.

MIXED VEGETABLE MEDLEY SOUP

1 tablespoon olive oil, chicken fat, or butter
1 onion, peeled and diced
2 garlic cloves, peeled and minced
1 (16-ounce) bag frozen mixed vegetables (any type)
1 (15-ounce) can diced tomatoes, undrained
4 cups chicken or vegetable stock, or water
½ teaspoon dried oregano or ½ tablespoon fresh
½ teaspoon dried basil or 3 to 4 leaves fresh basil, minced
1 teaspoon sea salt
Freshly ground black pepper
Fresh parsley sprigs

Preparation:

1. In a large pot, heat oil and sauté onions 2 to 3 minutes.
2. Add garlic and mixed vegetables, and sauté 1 to 2 minutes.
3. Add tomatoes, stock, oregano, basil, and salt.
4. Cover and cook on medium heat 10 to 12 minutes.
5. Add pepper to taste, and continue cooking 1 to 2 minutes.
6. Garnish each bowl of soup with a sprig of fresh parsley.

LENTILS WITH SPINACH AND SAUSAGE

1 bag frozen spinach or ½ bunch fresh spinach, cleaned and chopped

2 to 3 frozen sausage links (turkey, chicken, pork, etc.), thawed and diced

1 tablespoon olive oil

2 garlic cloves, peeled and minced

1 onion, peeled and diced

2 tablespoons fresh thyme leaves

1 (15-ounce) can brown, green, or black lentils, rinsed and drained

3½ cups chicken stock or water

2 bay leaves

1 teaspoon sea salt

Fresh parsley, minced

Preparation:

1. Remove spinach and sausage links from the freezer and thaw.
2. In a large pot, heat oil and sauté garlic and onions 1 to 2 minutes.
3. Add spinach and cook 2 to 3 minutes.
4. Add thyme, lentils, chicken stock, bay leaves, and sea salt.
5. Bring to a boil, cover, and simmer on low 15 to 20 minutes.
6. Remove and discard bay leaves.
7. Garnish with fresh parsley.

NOT SO CHIILLY CHILI

1 tablespoon olive oil
1 large onion, peeled and diced
3 garlic cloves, peeled and minced
1 teaspoon cumin
½ teaspoon coriander
2 frozen turkey, beef, or bison burgers, thawed and chopped into small pieces OR 1/2 pound ground pastured turkey meat
1 red pepper, seeded and diced
1 jalapeño pepper, seeded and diced
1 (15-ounce) can diced tomatoes, undrained
1½ cups cooked pinto beans or 1 (15-ounce) can pinto beans, rinsed and drained
½ teaspoon sea salt
Freshly ground black pepper
1 to 2 dashes cayenne pepper
Raw milk cheddar cheese, grated
1 tablespoon chives, minced (can use scallion)

Preparation:

1. In a deep frying pan or pot, heat oil and sauté onions and garlic 2 to 3 minutes.
2. Add cumin, coriander, and ground turkey pieces.
3. Add red pepper, jalapeño pepper, tomatoes, beans, salt, pepper to taste, and cayenne pepper.
4. Cover and cook on medium heat for 20 to 25 minutes.
5. Garnish with cheese and chives.

DELUXE BURGERS

Frozen pastured or organic burger patties (turkey, beef, buffalo or chicken), one per person
1 small onion, peeled and cut in thin crescents
2 to 3 button or cremini mushrooms, thinly sliced
1 tablespoon grass-fed butter or other fat
Sea salt
Raw milk Cheddar cheese or Monterey Jack (optional)
Whole grain burger buns (one per person) or whole grain bread slices (two per person)
Pickles, thinly sliced
Prepared stone ground mustard
Ketchup
Mayonnaise

Preparation:

1. Take burgers out of the freezer and thaw.
2. In a skillet, sauté onions and mushrooms in butter until soft and wilted.
3. Add a pinch or two of sea salt.
4. Remove sautéed vegetables and set aside.
5. Fry burger patties over medium-low heat.
6. Cover and cook 2 to 3 minutes.
7. Flip over, top with cheese (optional), cover, and cook an additional 2 to 3 minutes.
8. Lay cooked burger on bun or bread and top with onions, mushrooms, and 2 or 3 three pickle slices.
9. Smear your favorite condiments (ketchup, mustard, mayo) or a combination of all three on underside of top bun.

SASSY SHRIMP AND VEGETABLE STIR FRY WITH UDON NOODLES

8 to 10 ounces frozen shrimp (can use fresh shrimp, peeled and deveined)
1 (8-ounce) package udon noodles
1 onion, peeled and thinly sliced
2 garlic cloves, peeled and minced
1-inch ginger root, cut into matchsticks
1/3 cup chicken or fish stock, or water
2 carrots, thinly cut on the diagonal
½ head broccoli florets and stem (cut stem into ½-inch rounds)
½ tablespoon shoyu (naturally fermented soy sauce)
1 tablespoon toasted sesame oil
2 teaspoons maple syrup (or other liquid sweetener)
2 to 3 scallions, minced

Preparation:

1. Remove shrimp from the freezer and set on the counter to thaw.
2. Bring pot of water to boil, and cook udon noodles according to package directions.
3. Put onions, garlic, ginger, and stock in a sauté pan, and cook 2 to 3 minutes.
4. Add carrots and broccoli stems. Cover and cook 2 to 3 minutes.
5. Add broccoli florets and shrimp; cover.
6. Combine shoyu, sesame oil, and maple syrup, and add to the pan.
7. Cook 3 to 5 minutes or until shrimp are cooked and broccoli florets are bright green.
8. Dish out stir-fry on top of cooked udon noodles and garnish with minced scallions.

SIMPLE BERRY SORBETS

2 (8-ounce) bags frozen strawberries, blackberries, blueberries, cherries, or raspberries or 2 pints fresh berries, washed, patted dry, and frozen in freezer-safe bags

3 to 4 tablespoons grape jam (or other fruit preserves)

Preparation:

1. Remove frozen berries from the freezer and thaw 5 to 10 minutes or until slightly softened.
2. Place into a food processor or blender with fruit jam and quickly puree until smooth and creamy.
3. Serve immediately or refreeze and serve anytime.

PEACHES AND CREAM

2 (8-ounce) bags frozen peaches

½ cup cream

¼ cup beet sugar or other granulated sugar

Preparation:

1. Remove frozen peaches from the freezer and thaw 2 to 3 minutes.
2. While peaches are thawing slightly, combine sugar and cream.
3. Place peaches and cream into the food processor or blender and puree until smooth and creamy.
4. Serve immediately or refreeze and serve anytime.

Chapter 12

LIFESTYLE STRATEGIES OF THE HEALTHY & FABULOUS!

Frequent travel has taught me how to successfully navigate my way around our country's compromised food supply – even if I'm stranded at an airport! I saved this chapter for last because I wanted you to experiment cooking in your own kitchen before rushing out to a local restaurant for meals. Now that you have toiled and boiled and chopped your way through many delicious recipes, you may have a better understanding of what wholesome food could look and taste like.

People often erroneously believe that taking responsibility for their health means they can no longer enjoy eating out at restaurants, social gatherings, or other functions without suffering gustatory guilt. This couldn't be further from the truth. All we need to do now is take some home-cooking knowledge and apply it to meals outside the home. It's time to put down the knife and back away from the cutting board, we're heading out for some fun eating adventures.

TASTY TRAVELS

Eating, for me, is just as high a priority as finding shelter. I certainly would *not* plan a trip without figuring out, beforehand, where I was going lay my sleepy head for the night! As a conscious eater, before traveling, I do food research too. I'm not the kind of person who accidentally shows up in Podunk, USA, and plops myself down into any old restaurant for a meal. My travel itinerary always includes eating the best quality food available. Once I know my needs for food and shelter are met, I can truly relax and enjoy the destination.

Thanks to the internet, locating great food is practically effortless. It's as simple as entering the name of the city where you are headed plus the words, "local, seasonal, organic, naturally raised foods, restaurants." If there is something in that area it will pop up in an article, website, or blog. You could also go to localharvest.org or other "Resource" in the back of this book, and enter the zip code or city to help you find farmer's markets, grocery stores, and restaurants. On my website, there is a travel vlog (video blog) called Eating America! I actively seek out and showcase local, seasonal, organic, and naturally raised food in restaurants, farmers markets, CSA's, and more. Just type the name of the city or state that you are traveling to into the "search bar," and if we've been there, it'll show up.

This little bit of detective work makes discovering new places a yummy experience instead of a frantic search for food after arriving famished from a long day of traveling. You'll soon notice that once food becomes a priority, it's pretty darn easy to eat well no matter where you are.

You may be surprised to learn how many restaurants and chefs are sourcing high quality ingredients and they are proud of it – they boldly showcase local farmers and artisanal food producers on their menus. Savvy chefs and restaurateurs purchase from people who care about the products they create. For example, you may see something like this on a menu: "Appearing at Big Bob's diner, Martin Farms pastured chicken,

Stoneledge Farms Heirloom Tomatoes, and Squiggly Piggly Farms Heritage Bacon." It seems like farmers are the new rock stars!

If you don't have access to the internet, try the old fashioned way of digging up information: call the hotel, inn, or place where you are staying and ask if they know of any local, natural, seasonal restaurants, or health-food stores in the area. The local town-folk may know where to get the best homegrown, fresh, and natural products.

I love exploring new places and savoring local, seasonal, and indigenous ingredients. As an added bonus, eating locally grown food helps my body become physically acclimated to each new environment and eases the effects of jet lag and general fatigue from traveling. For example, I live in NYC, which has a temperate climate. If I were traveling to Costa Rica or some other tropical climate, upon arrival, I would need to eat the food growing in that area of the world to help rebalance my body. Eating locally in Costa Rica includes more fish and coconuts, as well as tropical fruits and other foods that help cool the body internally and keep it naturally balanced in the sweltering heat.

HOTEL, MOTEL, HOLIDAY INN...

Clients sometimes tell me that they don't have the option of leaving the hotel due to seminars, meetings, and other business obligations. In that case, it's imperative to check out the hotel restaurant menu before arriving. Many hotels have restaurants with great food on their menus. Some offer international fare for people traveling from all over the world.

If the hotel doesn't provide any quality food, or doesn't have a restaurant on site, ask if they have a room with a kitchenette. If yes, bring some simple travelling food: a small Ziploc baggie filled with rolled oats, dried fruit, and nuts and seeds (trail mix). With these few ingredients you can prepare a nourishing breakfast in your room.

If you don't want to travel with food, you could always find something to eat somewhere. This is America for gosh sakes! When I worked for MTV/VH1, I remember getting off the plane and driving directly to the nearest Whole Foods or natural foods market to stock up on eggs, bread, oats, butter, yogurt, and snacks like hummus before going to my hotel. I simply stored that stuff inside the small refrigerator in the hotel room.

If you do not have a room with a kitchenette and/or stove, you can still make a variety of foods in the coffee machine. Yes, that's right; I said, "in the coffee machine." To prepare basic oatmeal, we only need hot water. The same goes for soft-boiled eggs. You can acquire this magical cooking liquid by running the coffee machine without adding coffee. Voila! You've got hot water. For oatmeal, pour the hot water on top of rolled oats and let it sit covered overnight. In the morning pour a little more hot water on top, add some trail mix, and a dab of yogurt, and you've got a nourishing breakfast. To soft-boil an egg, fill a coffee cup with hot water and let the egg sit in it for 3 to 5 minutes. Change the water 3 to 4 times to achieve desired consistency. The longer you continue adding hot water, the more the egg cooks and the firmer it will be. Or you can drink the eggs "Rocky-style"; gulped down raw. Bleachhh! Not my favorite way to eat eggs. And, I can't believe I'm going to tell you this; but, you could even fry an egg on top of the coffee pot heating element (although not recommended, and very messy). By sharing that last tidbit of coffee pot cooking knowledge with you, I think I may have just been banned from every hotel in America.

RESTAURANT ORDERING

Eating in restaurants can seem a bit challenging for some folks; but once you get the hang of it, it's as easy as warm apple pie with a dollop of vanilla ice-cream on top. That's pretty darn easy, and delicious, too!

Keep in mind that most restaurants will accommodate patrons to ensure their meal is enjoyable. If you need your meal prepared in a specific way, don't hesitate to ask – they want to make you happy. If you have a pleasurable experience at a restaurant, you will likely return again and again.

There is a "health-oriented" restaurant located in the New York City neighborhood where I live. The kitchen notoriously undercooks the daily vegetables. And, the truth is, I cannot stomach raw broccoli and cauliflower. Ugh! I simply ask the server if my vegetables can be prepared "well done." In doing so, I get to enjoy a delicious easily digestible meal and they get a happy customer! Ask and ye shall receive.

Another thing to be aware of is that most restaurant portions are HUGE and may not be appropriately sized for your body. I've realized that some restaurant meals can be least twice the size of what I would normally eat at home. Knowing that, I do not order a full meal (appetizer and entrée plus a dessert) unless I'm eating at a high-end French restaurant where the portions are no bigger than a mere mouthful. That's probably the real reason how those French gals stay so darn thin. Portion control, baby!

If you live in a temperate climate, order a meal that is predominantly plant based with smaller amounts of animal protein (4 to 6 ounces, depending, of course, on your physical needs). Refer to the "Back to The Basics" chapter to get an idea of what a meal could look like. It's not uncommon for restaurants to serve 12 to 16 ounce steaks or other animal proteins and potatoes the size of Plymouth Rock. That may be appropriate for a linebacker, but not so good for little ole' me or you. How many times have you gone out to dinner and returned home, gingerly rubbing your bloated belly, saying, "Boy, am I stuffed. I feel like I'm about to give birth to a baby orca!" Okay, maybe you don't say exactly that, but something along those lines. Overstuffing ourselves happens all the time and may keep happening until we make the conscious connection that the amount of food piled on the plate may be more than our body needs.

To remedy this dilemma, I simply order an appetizer and then split a main meal with whomever I'm dining, or take half the entrée home. And, I *always* split a dessert. My body doesn't feel good or work well when it's overloaded with sugary sweets. Does yours?

It is easy to get healthful portions of vegetables and smaller portions of animal proteins in many Asian-influenced restaurants like Chinese, Japanese, Korean, Thai, and Vietnamese. Italian, Indian, Pakistani, French, American, Greek, Mexican, Kosher, Middle Eastern, and Spanish, usually serve some type of good quality carbohydrate like couscous, bulgur, rice, oats, beans, legumes, and a nice variety of cooked vegetables and raw salads.

Scan the menu to discern if there are any high quality animal foods that are organically grown, grass fed, pastured, antibiotic-free, or wild. These are better choices than factory-farmed animals. And, as mentioned earlier, restaurants sourcing good quality ingredients usually state it clearly on the menu.

If you are stranded without any good food options at a restaurant or other eatery that has no "naturally raised" products, don't sweat it. Just eat from a little lower on the food chain. Pesticides and chemicals accumulate more the higher up you go on the food chain – animal meats and dairy products may be the biggest offenders on a menu. In that case, choose something that is mostly, or all, vegetarian like soups, salads, some appetizers, and side dishes. And, if the majority of your food intake is the best quality, a little bit of poor quality food isn't going to harm you. Do the best you can most often and don't fret. The body can handle small amounts of toxins and pesticide residues – it's when our system becomes overburdened with excessive amounts that trouble arises.

Eating out at restaurants is a lot of fun, especially when you feel good about the food you're ingesting. Give yourself a break, get out of the house (not every night, of course) and let someone else do the cooking, and the dirty dishes, too.

SAVORY SOCIALIZING

I knew a woman who refused to attend parties and social gatherings because she didn't want to partake in any of the food being served. It was difficult for her to be around food she didn't want to eat. She was so intently focused on eating only her own food and/or food from specific health food restaurants that she never veered from her rigid eating regimen. Needless to say, she was one of the unhealthiest people I have ever known. Socially removed and physically detached, she was unable to be in the world in a functional way.

I saw a bit of myself in her (although not to that extreme) in my early thirties when I was strictly macrobiotic and then vegan. I recall refusing to eat food with my family at Thanksgiving and Christmas for a few years because I thought food was the only source of true nourishment.

Food is certainly a big part of healing because it creates our physical body. But, physical food is *not* the only thing needed to heal. We need a combination of mind, body, and spirit. And, you can't get that on a sandwich.

For example, a holiday meal prepared with pesticide-laden food but infused with the love of a family member who is cooking it, may be a better choice than a "clean" meal prepared with negative emotions and/or eaten alone. Socializing with loved ones can help support our spiritual and emotional growth. Besides it's not the *one* piece of sugary chocolate cake, or bowl of genetically modified corn chips, or cheap factory-farmed meat at the party that can harm us, it's the things we do consistently on a daily basis. If you're eating the best quality food most often, you can have a few unnaturally raised products, and it may not have such a detrimental effect. Unless, of course, you heap a big pile of guilt on top of your plate too.

If you are concerned about the food at the party, you could bring a dish that is lovingly prepared and made with good ingredients. The host may appreciate your gesture, and you'll know exactly what you're eating. It's a win-win situation.

The bottom line -- eat great quality products as often as possible and remember to enjoy your food and the people around you, too. This is surely a recipe for diet and lifestyle success.

Wherever you are, and whatever social environment you find yourself in, always remember that you are your greatest asset and you are worth it!

FOOD RESOURCES

ALVARADO STREET BAKERY
Phone: (707) 585-3293
www.alvaradostreetbakery.com
Whole grain bread products

AMAZON.com
http://www.amazon.com
Online retailer for food and kitchen products

COLEMAN NATURAL MEATS
http://www.colemannatural.com
Organic, naturally raised meats

DIAMOND ORGANICS
800-922-2396
www.diamondorganics.com
Organic produce and meats

EAT WELL GUIDE
www.eatwellguide.org
Directory of naturally raised products

EAT WILD
http://eatwild.com
Grass-fed animals products

EDEN FOODS
888-424-EDEN (3336)
www.edenfoods.com
Organic food products

FOODIELINK
http://www.foodielink.com
Connecting foodies with great food

GOLDMINE NATURAL FOODS
800-475-FOOD (3663)
http://www.goldminenaturalfoods.com
Organic foods and other products

KUSHI INSTITUTE STORE
800-645-8744
www.kushistore.com
Macrobiotic specialty items

LOCAL HARVEST
http://www.localharvest.org
Locate farmer's markets, CSAs, organic restaurants

AMERICAN GRASS FED BEEF
http://blog.americangrassfedbeef.com
recipes, information

MAINE COAST SEA VEGETABLES

207-565-2907

www.seaveg.com

Certified organic sea vegetables

RODALE INSTITUTE FARM LOCATOR

www.newfarm.org/farmlocator

Find organic farms

NIMAN RANCH

www.nimanranch.com

Toll Free 866-808-0340

Naturally raised meats

SUSTAINABLE TABLE

http://www.sustainabletable.org

Locate sustainable food

NATURAL RESOURCES DEFENSE COUNCIL

www.nrdc.org

ORGANIC CONSUMERS ASSOCIATION

www.organicconsumers.org

Promotes food safety and organic farming

SOUTH RIVER MISO

413-369-4057

www.southrivermiso.com

Organic miso products

TRADER JOES MARKET

www.traderjoes.com

Retailer of natural and organic products

WHOLE FOODS MARKET

www.wholefoodsmarket.com

Retailer of natural and organic products

WILD BY NATURE MARKET

http://www.wildnature.com

Retailer of natural and organic products

About The Author

Andrea Beaman is a natural foods chef, diet and lifestyle coach, and television host, with a passion for teaching people about sustainable eating and living. Successfully healing her *incurable* thyroid disease with health-promoting foods, exercise and natural therapies was the catalyst that transformed her health, life and profession.

Andrea was a contestant on Bravo's hit reality TV show, Top Chef (season 1). She is a regularly featured food and health expert on CBS News, and has appeared on Barbara Walters, The View, Emeril Live and Whole Living on Martha Stewart Radio. She hosts the *Award Nominated,* Fed UP! A cooking show that educates viewers how to cook for, and cure, bodily ailments. She maintains www.AndreaBeaman.com, her personal website that offers delicious recipes, fun video blogs, DVDs, personal health coaching, books, and other health-related information.

Andrea teaches at The Institute For Integrative Nutrition, the Natural Gourmet Cooking School, James Beard House, The Open Center, and other venues around the country to over 2000 students annually. Her high energy cooking classes and health seminars reach a wide base of clients and students. She makes learning about health, food, and positive lifestyle activities, a joy for everyone.

ANDREA BEAMAN BOOKS AND PRODUCTS

www.AndreaBeaman.com

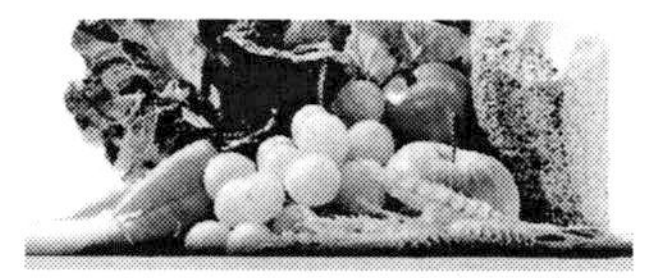

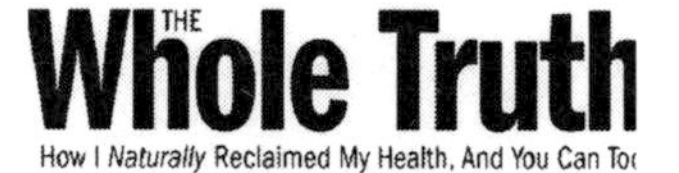

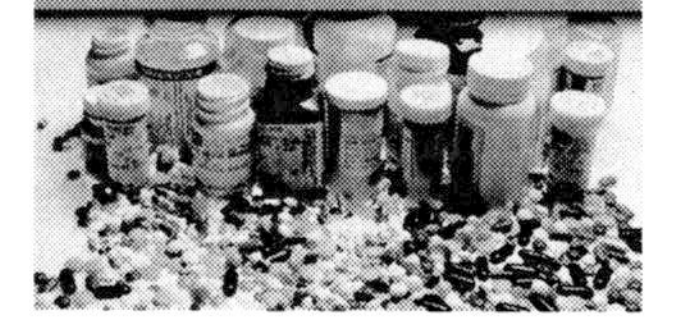

The Whole Truth How I Naturally Reclaimed My Health & You Can Too!
Retail $14.95

Check out Andrea's inspirational self-healing memoir that reveals eye-opening information about modern medical practices, and how sickness is a BIG business! The Whole Truth, How I Naturally Reclaimed My Health, provides useful tools to help readers begin their own healing journey. This is a must-read for anyone seeking health.

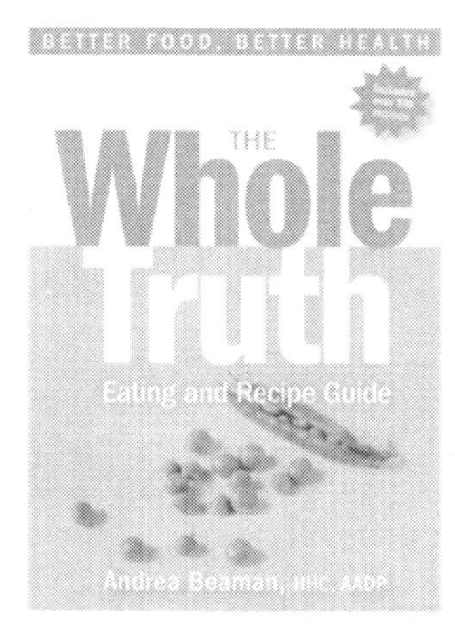

The Whole Truth Eating and Recipe Guide – Better Food, Better Health
Retail $19.95

The Whole Truth Eating and Recipe Guide presents an understanding of food and its effect on long-term health and vitality. With this practical knowledge, vibrant health and an ideal weight can easily be achieved without restrictive dieting. Included in this enlightening and humorous guide are more than 100 delicious recipes.

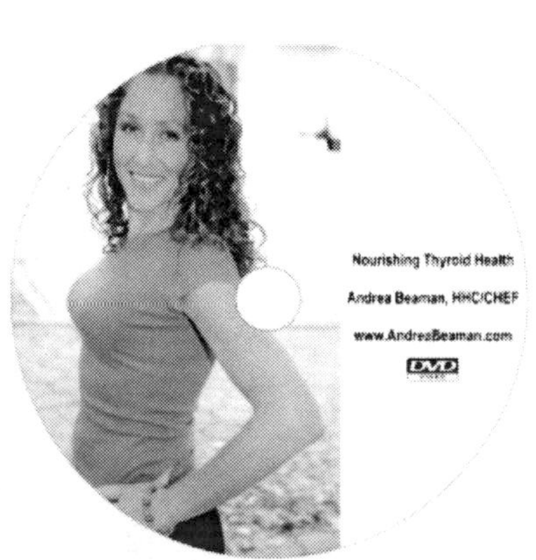

Nourishing Thyroid Health
Retail $24.99

Join Andrea in this educational and entertaining video as she shares the steps she took to successfully heal her own debilitating Thyroid disease and how you can, too. From environmental factors, to food choices, and emotional healing, this DVD has what you need to begin healing your thyroid right now!

RECIPE INDEX

A

ASPARAGUS SOUP, 208

B

BAKED CHICKEN, 133
BAKED CHICKEN & ROSEMARY-
ROASTED POTATOES, 133
BASIC BLACK BEANS, 156
BASIC BROWN RICE, 114
BASIC CHICKEN STOCK, 98
BASIC VEGETABLE STOCK, 102
BEAN SALAD, 159
BEAN STEW, 195, 197
BEANS, 156, 159, 195, 197
BEEF, 202
BEEF STEW, 202
BEEF STOCK, 101
BERRY SORBETS, 216
BLACK BEAN SOUP, 160
BLACK BEANS, 156, 159
BLACKBERRIES, 216
BLACK-EYED PEA SOUP, 118
SOUP, 118
BLACK-EYED PEAS, 112, 118, 119, 198
BLACK-EYED PEAS AND VEGETABLE
WRAP
WRAP, 119
BLACK-EYED PEAS WITH CHORIZO, 112
BLUEBERRIES, 216
BRAISED DUCK, 174
BRAISED RED CABBAGE AND KALE, 115
BREAKFAST PORRIDGE, 80
BROCCOLI, 134
BROWN BASMATI RICE, 146
BROWN RICE, 114
BRUSSELS SPROUTS, 179
BUFFALO, 200
BUFFALO CHILI, 200
BURGERS, 214

C

CACCIATORE, 138
CANNELINI BEANS, 141, 197
CARAMELIZED ONION SOUP, 182
CARROTS, 134
CHEESE AND VEGGIE OMELET, 136
CHERRIES, 216
CHICKEN, 138, 196
CHICKEN CACCIATORE, 138
CHICKEN LIVER, 135
CHICKEN LIVER PÂTÉ, 135
CHICKEN SALAD, 140
CHICKEN SAUSAGE, 212
CHICKEN SOUP, 196
CHICKEN STOCK, 98
CHILI, 190, 198, 200, 213
CHILI CON CARNE, 198
CHINESE CABBAGE SALAD, 176
CHORIZO, 112
CHOWDER, 170, 210
CHUNKY CHICKEN SOUP, 196
COBBLER, 116
COCONUT RICE PUDDING, 153
COLLARD GREENS, 167
CONGEE, 82
CORN, 11, 30, 158, 210, 225
CORN CHOWDER, 210
CORNMEAL, 157
COUSCOUS, 163
COUSCOUS PORRIDGE
PORRIDGE, 166
CRACKED OATS, 84
CRACKLINS, 176
CRANBERRY DRESSING, 148
CREAMY ASPARAGUS SOUP, 208
CREAMY COCONUT RICE PUDDING, 153
CREAMY POLENTA AND FRIED EGGS, 92
CREAMY TURKEY CHOWDER, 170
CRISPY GARLIC CROUTONS, 141, 142
CROUTONS, 142
CURRIED CHICKEN SALAD, 140

D

DELUXE BURGERS, 214
DRESSING, 148
DRY ROASTED NUTS, 81
DUCK, 174, 181
DUCK BREAST, 176
DUCK FAT, 175
DUCK LIVER PÂTÉ, 181
DUCK STOCK, 99

E

EGGS, 88, 90, 92

F

FIVE-MINUTE MISO SOUP, 129
FLOUNDER, 124
FLUKE, 124
FRIED POLENTA SQUARES, 158
FRIED RICE, 120

G

GARLIC BREAD, 139
GARLIC CROUTONS, 142
GRAVY, 164, 171

H

HEARTY BEEF STEW, 202
HEARTY LENTIL STEW, 188
HEARTY ROASTED WINTER ROOTS, 178
HERBED GARLIC BREAD, 139
HERBED GRAVY, 164, 171
HOME FRIES, 137
HOMEMADE MAYO, 169
HOMEY HOME FRIES, 137
HOT OPENED TURKEY SANDWICHES
    WITH HERBED GRAVY, 171

K

KALE, 35, 141, 147
KAMUT ELBOW PASTA, 186
KIDNEY BEANS, 186, 198
KOMBU, 156

L

LAMB, 204
LEMON SOLE, 124
LENTIL AND VEGETABLE WRAP, 150
LENTIL SOUP, 152
LENTIL STEW
    SOUP, 188
LENTILS, 145, 150, 152, 212
LENTILS WITH SAUTÉED LEEKS,
    SPINACH, AND SAUSAGE, 145
LENTILS WITH SPINACH AND SAUSAGE,
    212
LIVER PÂTÉ, 181

M

MAGNIFICENT MINESTRONG, 186
    SOUP, 186
MAYONNAISE, 169
MINESTRONE
    SOUP, 186
MISO, 83, 129, 192, 194
MISO SALMON SOUP, 83
MISO SOUP, 129
MIXED VEGETABLE MEDLEY SOUP, 211
MUSHROOM SOUP, 180

N

NOODLES, 105
NORI, 174
NOT SO CHIILLY CHILI, 213
NUTS, 149

O

OATS & ALMONDS, 84
    PORRIDGE, 84
OATS & SAUSAGE, 85
OMELET, 136
    EGGS, 136
ONE-POT WILD SALMON STEW, 192
ONION SOUP, 182

P

PAN-SEARED DUCK BREAST & CHINESE
    CABBAGE SALAD WITH CRUNCHY
    CRACKLINS, 176

PASTA, 186
PASTA SALAD, 168
PÂTÉ, 135
PEA SOUP, 209
PEACHES, 217
PEACHES AND CREAM, 217
PINTO BEANS, 190, 200, 213
POACHED EGGS, 88
POLENTA, 92, 157, 158, 160
POLENTA AND FRIED EGGS, 92
POLENTA WITH SAUTÉED SHITAKE MUSHROOMS AND TURKEY SAUSAGE, 157
POPSICLES, 217
PORRIDGE, 80
PORRIDGE, 166

Q

QUICK-COOKING CHICKEN CACCIATORE, 138
QUICK-COOKING FRIED RICE, 120

R

RASPBERRIES, 216
RAVISHING ROLLED OATS PORRIDGE, 86
RED CABBAGE AND KALE, 115
RENDERED DUCK FAT, 175
RESOURCES, 227
RICE PUDDING, 153
ROASTED NUTS, 81
ROASTED TURKEY, 164
ROASTED TURKEY WITH HERBED GRAVY, 164
ROASTED WINTER ROOTS, 178
ROASTING NUTS, 149
ROLLED OATS
PORRIDGE, 86
ROOTS, 178
ROSEMARY ROASTED POTATOTES, 133

S

SALAD, 168
SALMON, 192
SALMON SOUP, 83
SALMON STEW, 192
SASSY SHRIMP AND VEGETABLE STIR FRY, 215
SAUSAGE, 85, 112, 145, 150, 157, 212
SAUTÉED BLACK-EYED PEAS AND VEGETABLE WRAP, 119
SAUTÉED BOK CHOY & CARROTS, 127
SAUTÉED BRUSSELS SPROUTS WITH CRANBERRIES, 179
SAUTÉED COLLARD GREENS WITH GARLIC, 167
SAVORY COUSCOUS PORRIDGE
PORRIDGE, 166
SAVORY OATS & SAUSAGE, 85
SAVORY RICE & OATS PORRIDGE, 114
SAVORY SHITAKE MUSHROOM SOUP, 180
SAVORY TURKEY CHILI, 190
SCRAMBLED EGGS CON VEGGIES, 90
SEA BASS, 194
SEA BASS SOUP WITH SOBA NOODLES, 194
SEASONAL BEAN SALAD IN LETTUCE CUPS, 159
SESAME-CRUSTED SOLE, 124
SHITAKE MUSHROOM SOUP, 180
SHITAKE MUSHROOMS, 157
SHRIMP, 151
SHRIMP AND VEGETABLE STIR FRY, 215
SILKY CORN CHOWDER, 210
SILKY LENTIL SOUP, 152
SIMPLE BERRY SORBETS, 216
SIMPLE BROWN BASMATI RICE, 146
SIMPLE SAUTÉED CARROTS AND BROCCOLI, 134
SIMPLE SOBA NOODLES, 126
SIRLOIN STEAK, 198
SLOW COOKER STOCK, 103
SOBA NOODLE, 128
SOBA NOODLE STIR-FRY
STIR FRY, 128
SOBA NOODLES, 126, 194
SOLE, 124
SORBETS, 216
SOUP, 152, 208, 209
SPICY BLACK BEAN SOUP WITH POLENTA CROUTONS, 160
SPRING PEA SOUP, 209
STEAK, 198
STEAMED WINTER VEGETABLES WITH TOASTED WALNUTS AND CRANBERRY DRESSING, 147
STEWED LAMB WITH APRICOTS, 204
STIR FRY, 215
STIR-FRIED SHRIMP, RICE, AND VEGETABLES, 151
STIR-FRY, 128, 151
STOCK, 98, 99, 100, 101

STRAWBERRIES, 216
SUMMER VEGETABLES AND BEAN STEW, 197

T

TAHINI NOODLES, 174
TAHINI NOODLES & BRAISED DUCK, 174
TEX-MEX CHILI CON CARNE, 198
TOASTING NUTS, 149
TOFU, 151
TURKEY, 164, 170
TURKEY AND PASTA SALAD, 168
TURKEY CHILI, 190
TURKEY CHOWDER, 170
TURKEY SALAD, 168
TURKEY SANDWICHES, 171
TURKEY SAUSAGE, 157
TURKEY STOCK, 100

U

UDON NOODLES, 174, 215

V

VEGETABLE SOUP, 211
VEGETABLE STOCK, 102
VEGETABLES AND BEAN STEW, 197

W

WHITE BEAN AND KALE SOUP, 141
WHITE BEAN STEW, 195
WHOLE GRAIN COUSCOUS WITH DRIED CRANBERRIES, 163
WHOLE GRAIN HERBED GARLIC BREAD, 139
WHOLE WHEAT COUS COUS, 163
WILD SALMON STEW, 192
WINTER COBBLER, 116
WINTER ROOTS, 178
WINTER WHITE BEAN STEW, 195
WRAPS, 150

CPSIA information can be obtained at www.ICGtesting.com
231338LV00002B/45/P

9 780977 869336